Genetics
& Your Health

A GUIDE for the
21st Century Family

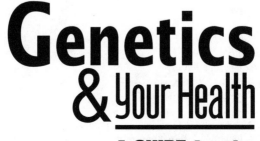

Genetics
& Your Health

A GUIDE for the
21st Century Family

Raye Lynn Alford, Ph.D., FACMG
Foreword by Robert E. Pollack, Ph.D.

MEDFORD

P R E S S

Genetics & Your Health
A Guide for the 21st Century Family

Library of Congress Cataloging-in-Publication Data

Alford, Raye Lynn, 1962-
    Genetics & Your Health : a guide for the 21st century family /
    Raye Lynn Alford.
        p.   cm.
    Includes bibliographical references and index.
    ISBN 0-9666748-2-0 (hardcover)   ISBN 0-9666748-1-2 (pbk.)
    1. Medical genetics--Popular works.   2. Human genetics--Popular
works.   I. Title.
RB155.A39   1999
616'.042--dc21   98-31950
                          CIP

Cover Design: Bette Tumasz
Book Design: Patricia F. Kirkbride
Index: Sharon Hughes

For Bobby and Othelia

Table of Contents

Foreword

About a year ago, a friend of mine was diagnosed with cancer of the prostate. As he was my own age and had pretty much my physical build and background, this news was unsettling, even threatening to me. Although I had no symptoms of prostate trouble, his diagnosis cast a vague shadow on me. That troubling feeling took specific form as soon as my friend told me how he had come to be diagnosed.

He had been to a doctor who advised him—on grounds I did not ask about—to have a blood sample tested for the amount of a chemical called Prostate-Specific Antigen, or PSA. PSA is prostate specific in the sense that only the prostate gland produces it. An excess of PSA in the blood is a sign of prostate cells that can turn—or have turned—into a malignancy of the gland.

Based on the results of his PSA-test, his doctor had recommended a biopsy of the prostate, an unpleasant procedure with a significant risk of lasting side-effects, also unpleasant. He had had the biopsy taken, and in that bit of tissue from the well of his body were, indeed, just the sort of malignant cells that, if left alone for long, would have spread into a serious, even life-threatening illness.

Once he had the requisite operation to remove the diseased tissue, he became in his recovery an implacable recommender of the PSA-test. He followed his male friends around, shameless in his devotion to the idea that, like him, our choice was either to have the test done, or die of cancer. He would recognize no middle ground in which the absence of symptoms and the risk of side-effects justified not having the test done.

I took refuge in my habits as a scientist and looked up the statistics on this test. I found that about one time in three, a positive test followed by biopsy does not reveal any abnormality whatsoever, and of the positive tests that are accompanied by abnormal biopsies, only about one in ten are malignant changes. The others are milder, and while they may eventually lead to malignancy, they also may not. With these facts in mind, and mindful as well of the possible side-effects of a biopsy, I simply could not decide what to do.

I took myself to my doctor. She heard me out and decided that I was already so agitated that the PSA test ought to be done, if only to ease the strain of it all. She also agreed on two prerequisites: first, that she would remain my advisor on all subsequent decisions should the test prove positive, and second, that given the high level of false-positives and the very low frequency of real malignancies found on biopsy, if the PSA-test were positive and I still chose not to have a biopsy, she would support that decision.

I had the test done. The results were negative, and so there is nothing more to say about my prostate, except this. I have rarely been so frightened in my life, as in those days when I was waiting for the results of this test. It is that fear which this wonderful book hopes to allay—and does.

Genetics & Your Health is the prospective patient's essential reference, the book each of us—man or woman, young or old—should have with us when we are in the position I was in. Regardless of how much we know about human genetics, molecular biology, or medicine, we are all in need of a calm guide when we are agitated by personal risk. This book is a book you should read now, while no one is asking you—or telling you—that there is any reason to have any diagnostic test done at all.

In time, as the techniques of molecular diagnosis and prognosis get ever more efficient and as they cover an ever larger number of diseases and conditions, the chances approach certainty that one day you will be asked or told to have such a test. At that moment, you will be glad, I am sure, that you have already read this book and have it at hand.

Robert E. Pollack, Ph.D.
Professor of Biological Sciences
Columbia University

Robert Pollack worked for several years with James Watson, the co-discoverer of DNA's structure, at Cold Spring Harbor Laboratory. For many years a professor of biological sciences at Columbia University, he also served as dean of Columbia College through much of the 1980s. A recent winner of a Guggenheim writing fellowship, he now divides his time between New York City and Vermont. He is the author of Signs of Life: The Language and Meanings of DNA. *Boston: Houghton Mifflin, 1995.*

Acknowledgments

Grateful acknowledgment is extended to the following individuals: to David Nelson, Ph.D. for critical evaluation of the manuscript; to Bobby R. Alford, M.D., Scott Alford, and Lauren Hagan for their insight, perspective, and comments on the manuscript; to Dan Arnold and Naomi Broering for their devoted assistance and advice; to Robert Pollack for his Foreword and suggestions; to Walter Wager; to Dr. Joshua Lederberg; to Tom Hogan Sr., John Bryans, Dorothy Pike, Pat Palatucci, Heide Dengler, Bette Tumasz, Patricia F. Kirkbride, Rhonda Forbes, Judy Bouchard, Tom Hogan Jr., Heather Rudolph, and everyone else at Plexus Publishing, Inc. for their commitment to this project; and to my friends and family for their support, encouragement, and vision.

Introduction

In recent years, scientists have learned a lot about the genetic factors that affect human health. Hundreds of human genetic conditions have been characterized in detail, but the genetic factors involved in so many more have yet to be understood. To that end, researchers are actively pursuing new knowledge about genetics. In labs all over the world, scientists are locating, isolating, and characterizing genes. Genes are basic units of inheritance that contribute to the characteristics of every living thing. Finding a gene is an important discovery because it gives scientists a new tool for studying the growth, development, and function of all kinds of biological organisms.

The recent successes of genetic research are proving to have implications for mankind that reach far beyond the laboratory. Genetic advances are being applied to routine medical practice at an unprecedented rate. Almost daily, genetic discoveries provide doctors and patients with better ways to diagnose, treat, or prevent illness. Genetic science is also finding its way into our courtrooms as evidence in criminal proceedings and into our history books confirming or refuting accounts of historical events.

Because of the rapidly growing applications of genetics, public interest in genetic research has increased steadily. Reports of scientific inquiry geared toward unraveling the mysteries of our DNA and how genes affect our growth, development, and health have become commonplace. Can you remember the last time you picked up a newspaper or turned on the television and saw a report about DNA testing or the identification of a gene responsible for a particular trait or disease? It probably wasn't very long ago.

Much of the rapid progress and prominent publicity of genetic research is due to the success of the largest single project ever undertaken in the biological sciences, the Human Genome Project. The Human Genome Project is an internationally organized research effort designed to systematically and completely decipher the genetic information of man and several other organisms. The project focuses on gene discovery, technological advancement, application of findings to medicine and evaluation of ethical, legal, and social issues associated with genetic science.

Prior to the Human Genome Project, looking for the genetic cause of an illness was very difficult because there were few clues about how to locate any particular gene. Now, researchers have a detailed map of the genetic content of man. This genetic road map facilitates the search for genes and the detection of disease-causing genetic alterations. Advances in laboratory technologies have also helped make the search for genes faster and more efficient than ever before. Researchers are currently working toward deciphering the smallest details of the genetic information of man. So far, the scientific goals of the Human Genome Project are being met on or ahead of schedule, and complete discovery of the genetic information of man is anticipated by the year 2003.

Already, genetic research has refined our perceptions about the role genes play in many human traits. Genetic research has brought scientists and doctors a deeper knowledge of how the human body is built, how it functions, and what genetic factors contribute to human illness. Genetic science has touched all aspects of medicine, improving our understanding and management of heart disease; shedding light on the causes of cystic fibrosis, sickle cell anemia, and muscular dystrophy; and opening doors to new treatments for cancer and birth defects.

In addition to the goals of the Human Genome Project for discovering the genes of man, scientific analysis of genes from organisms such as bacteria, yeast, worms, fruit flies, and mice has advanced our understanding of what genes do. These and other organisms, with short reproductive times and easily studied tissues, give scientists important model systems in which to study how genes mediate the growth, development, and health of an individual. Such model systems are vital to basic research and the development of safe, effective treatment methods for all types of illnesses—not just genetic ones.

There are many human illnesses that are known to have a strong genetic component. It is estimated that at least 30 to 50 percent of childhood and 10 percent of adult hospital admissions involve disorders that are strongly influenced by genes. Many genetic diseases are fairly common. Conditions such as muscular dystrophy, cystic fibrosis, sickle cell anemia, and thalassemia affect millions of people worldwide. The thousands of different genetic conditions can vary widely in their symptoms and impact on the health of the affected individual. Some genetic conditions may go almost completely unnoticed while others may be extremely debilitating. Some genetic diseases are apparent at birth and others may not become evident until late in life. Some genetic diseases can be influenced greatly by diet and environment.

For many genetic diseases and traits, research has already discovered the genes involved. As we learn more about the genetic influences on diabetes, multiple sclerosis, heart disease, hypertension, depression, mental retardation, and many other common conditions, most of us are likely to be influenced in some direct way by genetic science.

With the biochemical and genetic causes of many human diseases now defined, scientists are able to develop new strategies for the rapid and precise diagnosis of genetic disease. As a result, doctors are able to test for and diagnose many genetic diseases in the laboratory. It is expected that, given the current pace of genetic research, the number of diseases for which genetic testing is available will continue to increase rapidly.

Sometimes the diagnostic capabilities of genetic testing are used to confirm the suspicion of an illness in a patient with characteristic symptoms. In other cases, genetic testing can detect a predisposition to developing an illness later in life. In fact, the probability of developing some diseases can now be assessed well before symptoms appear in a patient or even before birth.

The ability to diagnose clinical disease accurately has been an important aspect of medical practice for centuries. In this context, genetic testing is comparable to other types of medical tests. However, the ability to detect genetic diseases presymptomatically or prenatally or to identify healthy carriers of genetic diseases who are at risk for having children affected by a disease is fairly new. Benefits of genetic testing can include improved diagnosis of disease, improved management of patients and their families, possible reduction in disease occurrence, and, ultimately, effective treatments or even cures.

For example, consider the ability to test, at a young age, for the likelihood that an individual might develop a certain type of cancer. If this information could be used to more effectively manage at-risk individuals through early detection, successful treatment, extension of life expectancy, and improvement in the quality of life, how many people would be interested in the technology? Imagine the possibilities if effective treatments are found for diseases such as Alzheimer's disease, diabetes, and heart disease. If methods become available to determine exactly who will need treatment and when it should begin, early intervention might actually be able to reduce the burden of many diseases in the future.

Herein lies what is perhaps the greatest promise of genetic research: more effective management of human illnesses. This hope stems from the growing knowledge about the basic functions of cells. In the same way that understanding how and why a car engine is put together is necessary to being able to fix one, understanding which genes are required by a cell for a particular function of the body is vital if we are to learn how differences in genes cause health problems. Through this knowledge, we gain insight for problem solving.

Currently, treatments for genetic diseases take many forms, from drug therapies to dietary intervention to surgery. It is likely that many of the same principles will be applied in the future. And with the knowledge gained from genetic research, new approaches such as gene therapy are being developed to combat particularly difficult therapeutic problems. However, these new abilities raise a number of ethical, legal, and social issues.

Perhaps the greatest fear of genetic research is that, with this rapid progression of science into uncharted territory, challenging questions arise about how the new capabilities and technologies will be used. The societal debate over the applications of genetics to medicine must address concerns over privacy and confidentiality of genetic test results, fears of social stigmatization, protection from discrimination in employment or insurance, and avoidance of the misuse of genetic technologies and information. Like any other new technology, the risks, benefits, applications, and limitations of medical genetic technologies must be carefully explored and evaluated in order to optimize the capabilities and minimize the abuses.

Unfortunately, genetics is at an awkward stage, one in which the ability to predict diseases, in most instances, far precedes our ability to treat them. As such, we must work to develop fair and effective ways to balance the potential good of genetic science against the possible misuses.

To achieve this balance, we must work together as a society to share information and resolve concerns. As scientists, we must take steps to inform every individual about the important potential of genetic research. As citizens, we must consider all aspects of medical genetic technology including the potential applications of the science; its possible contributions to improving the welfare of all mankind; and the medical, social, and ethical limitations and risks associated with our new skills. We must all learn about the issues if we are to be able to separate fact from fiction.

Already, we are having to consider complicated questions such as how does all of this new genetic information help individuals, patients, and families? How should genetic information be used? Who should have access to genetic information? How do we maximize the use of genetic knowledge for the treatment of disease? How do we manage the social and psychological implications of a genetic diagnosis? How do we protect ourselves against the potential for stigmatization and discrimination? What lasting effects will the application of medical genetics to health care have on individuals and society?

On a more personal level, the first time most people fully realize the impact of genetics on their own lives is when they are diagnosed with a genetic disease or when they are faced with a child or relative that has been diagnosed with a genetic disease. Under such difficult emotional circumstances, it can be challenging for patients and families to comprehend the complex information provided by doctors, nurses, and genetic counselors, especially if it is the first time they have ever considered the science of genetics and the implications surrounding a genetic diagnosis.

Making medical decisions under these conditions is very difficult, and since genetics is a very new science, most people went to school at a time when our understanding of it was primitive. As such, it can be a daunting task for individuals to consider the facts, assess their options, and draw conclusions about the correct course of action for them. Do not feel intimidated if you are easily confused by the subject—you are not alone.

In fact, many doctors today have not had formal training in the principles and practice of genetics. This is because many practicing physicians attended medical school before we had much knowledge about genetics. The genetic knowledge they have gained has most likely been acquired in much the same way that their patients have learned it—through self-education. As a result, doctors and patients alike can have many questions about genetics, its application to medicine, and the interpretation of genetic test results. Often, patients who conscientiously research their concerns and educate themselves about genetics will find that they know as much as their doctor does about the genetics of an illness that affects them.

Because genetic science is so new, there is a growing need for both public and professional education about genetic disease. An educated public is vital. Educating yourself as much as you can about the genetics of conditions that affect you and your family is the best way to take control of your own health and the health of your family. Educating physicians will be important if medical genetics is going to fulfill its potential impact on human health quickly. Physicians called clinical geneticists are often the most highly trained medical resource for patients with concerns about genetic disease. Genetic counselors are also a highly trained, vital resource for patients and families. These professionals are educated specifically in genetics and are trained to assist patients and families with their concerns about genetic illness.

For the thousands of people who already participate in genetic testing procedures each year, gaining a practical understanding of genetics is of great interest. As the number of illnesses for which genetic testing is available grows, medical genetics is likely to touch the lives of many thousands more of us, especially as treatment options become available for currently incurable diseases.

Genetic testing during pregnancy is also becoming more commonplace. More and more, couples are interested in learning about the genetic health of their unborn children. Genetic tests give couples the opportunity to ask specific questions, and for expectant parents, learning that their unborn child may have a genetic disease can obviously be very traumatic. Having the information contained within this book will help parents and families answer questions and gain confidence in the decisions they make.

The purpose of this book is to provide a basic education in genetic science and its applications to modern medical practice. Readers will acquire an understanding of the principles of genetics, the potential of genetics, the power of genetic testing, and ways to identify genetics professionals and genetics resources in your area. Readers will also learn about the applications of genetics, its importance to human health, and the ethical issues surrounding genetic testing and genetic research. This will facilitate interpreting genetic information seen in the news or provided by health-care professionals, taking advantage of medical resources available for the diagnosis and treatment of genetic disease, and understanding the impact and uses of genetic information.

The first chapters of this book provide a basic introduction to the science of genetics including a discussion of what genes are, where they are found, what purpose they serve, and how they work to influence our growth, development, and health. Next, readers learn how alterations in genes can cause disease and how genetic disease is passed from parent to child through generations. A brief introduction is given into the calculation of genetic risks. In this regard, Chapters 9 through 11 are the most scientifically challenging chapters of the book.

In later chapters, readers will find a discussion of the types of genetic tests that are available, when to consider a genetic test, and what important questions to ask when considering genetic testing. Readers are led through a discussion of the important potential of genetic science in human health. Finally, a discussion is presented on the applications of genetic research to medicine with special consideration of future developments that could provide options for treating or even curing diseases that have, up to now, been difficult to manage. The last chapters provide guidelines and resources for obtaining medical care, information, and support for medical genetics concerns.

While certain genetic diseases may be used to illustrate points, it is not the intent of this book to provide detailed information about specific diseases or give readers sufficient diagnostic or therapeutic insight to avoid the need for consultation with doctors, geneticists, or genetic counselors. It would not be possible to replace qualified genetic counseling or medical consultation in any book, and it is not the intent of this book to replace qualified medical genetics care.

Because genetics is a rapidly progressing science and new discoveries occur literally every day, it is best for anyone with concerns about a particular genetic disease to seek out qualified medical genetics care and obtain up-to-date information and guidance. The resources for genetics services are growing rapidly, and patients and families should be able to take advantage of the medical support that is available.

CHAPTER ONE

The Basics

The human body is a highly organized, complex structure made up of many different organs and tissues such as skin, muscle, bone, heart, eyes, ears, stomach, and liver. Each of these organs and tissues is made up of millions of microscopic components called cells. The cell is the basic building block of the body, and many millions of cells combine to make up the organs and tissues that combine to make up the body.

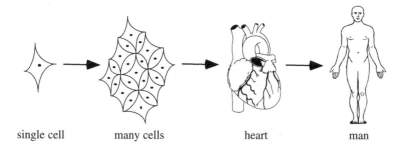

single cell   many cells   heart   man

FIGURE 1.1   A step-by-step diagram showing how single cells combine in groups to assemble organs, tissues, and bodies.

The different organs and tissues of the body each have their own sizes and shapes. Imagine for a moment the differences in the size and shape of your lungs, your heart, your brain, and your eyes. Each of these different organs and tissues is designed to perform highly specialized tasks. Your lungs allow you to breathe and get oxygen to your blood. Your heart beats to circulate the blood throughout your body. Your brain manages the conscious thoughts and movements and the unconscious functions of your body. Your eyes allow you to see.

The differences in structure and function of the organs and tissues of the body are possible because the cells that make them up have the ability to do very different things. One of the basic goals of biology is to understand how so many functionally distinct cells occur and what makes cells different enough to allow the diversity of structures, organs, and tissues.

To understand the differences in organs and tissues, we must first look at how all these different cell types arise. The billions of cells that make up the body arise during a complex process of growth and development. Each body starts as a single cell—a fertilized egg. This single cell is the result of a process called fertilization, which occurs when the sperm from the male and the egg from the female combine. After fertilization, the egg undergoes a process of cell division called "mitosis" in which the cell splits or divides to become two identical daughter cells. Mitosis continues throughout the growth and development of the body and results in cells dividing over and over again. Mitosis produces, from a single cell, all the billions of cells that make up the organs and tissues of the body.

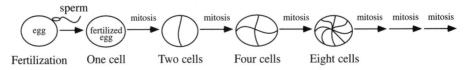

FIGURE 1.2 At conception, the egg is fertilized by the sperm. The fertilized egg then begins to divide by mitosis, resulting in all the cells of the body.

Normally, each fertilized egg starts out with all the genetic information that is needed to make a whole person. This genetic information is a collection of thousands of individual units called "genes." Taken together, all the cell's genes make up a sort of cellular library containing all of the reference information needed to tell a cell what to do and how to do it.

The genes in this library are inherited from one's parents at the time of fertilization through the sperm and the egg. Genes are organized on structures called "chromosomes." Physically, chromosomes can be visualized as tiny pieces of string. A human cell has forty-six chromosomes—or forty-six individual pieces of string.

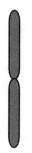

FIGURE 1.3   A chromosome. Human cells have forty-six chromosomes. Usually, chromosomes in cells are stretched out in long pieces like an unrolled ball of string. At the time of mitosis, the chromosomes condense into compact, tightly coiled, rod-shaped structures as drawn here. Throughout this book, chromosomes will be drawn in this condensed form, but remember that looking at a typical cell through a microscope will not reveal such a compact, visible picture of chromosomes.

In function, the chromosomes are the scaffolding that holds the genes—or the bookshelves in the genetic library. In this library, the genes are the books, the individual sets of instructions that provide the cell with the information necessary for building the components of the body.

Throughout the growth and development of a body, cells make an exact copy of each chromosome before every cell division. During mitosis, one copy of each of the duplicated chromosomes is assigned to the newly forming cells so that each daughter cell receives a complete set of the genetic information that was contained within its parent cell.

With the notable exception of red blood cells, all the cells of the body contain a complete set of the genes that we as individuals carry. As a result, examination of the genes from almost any cell of an individual can usually tell a doctor or scientist about the genes in all the other cells. For example, if a genetic test is performed on genes isolated from a few white blood cells called "lymphocytes" or a few skin cells called "fibroblasts," scientists can

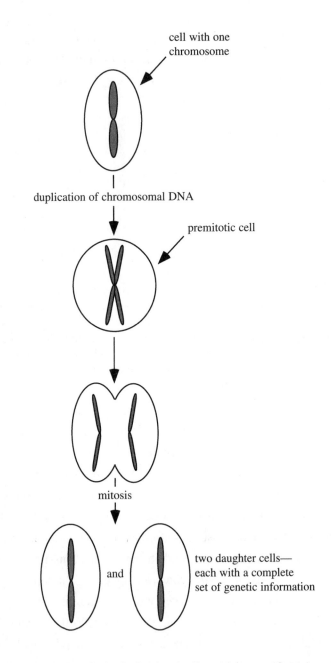

FIGURE 1.4   A step-by-step drawing of mitosis showing a cell containing one chromosome. Before mitosis, cells duplicate or make copies of all of their chromosomes. During mitosis, the duplicated chromosomes are divided up so that each of the new daughter cells receives one of each chromosome. After mitosis, each new daughter cell should contain a complete set of the genetic information that was contained in the parent cell.

usually learn about the genetic information of the whole individual. This is why a blood sample is generally sufficient for a genetic test, because the lymphocytes contain the same genetic information as the other cells of the body. Another good source of DNA for genetic testing is the buccal cells from the inside surface of one's cheek. These cells are easy to collect with a small, soft brush or a tongue depressor and, like lymphocytes, they generally contain the same genetic information as the other cells of the body.

Exceptions occur in certain disorders such as cancer where some cells of the body may carry a genetic mutation that is not found in other cells. This sometimes means that doctors must obtain a sample from a specific tissue in order to collect the particular cells affected by a genetic disease. In such cases, the collection of cells related only to the disease may improve a doctor's ability to identify the genetic alteration that has caused the illness.

So far, we have learned that the genes contained within the cell's genetic library provide the cell with a sort of owner's manual or instructions for carrying out the functions of the body. The cell uses the instructions encoded in the genes to make proteins. A protein is the functional representation of a gene's instructions. Proteins are the cellular workers responsible for performing specific tasks. The capabilities of these workers come from the information contained within the genes.

So the question arises, if, as a result of mitosis, all the cells of the body contain the same genetic information and if all cells use this genetic information to make proteins, shouldn't all cells be the same? The appearance of the different organs and tissues that exist in the body shows us that all cells are not the same. A tremendous amount of scientific research has been geared toward learning how the diversity in cellular function occurs.

What scientists have learned is that cells are different because each individual cell uses the genetic information in its own specialized way. All cells do not need all the proteins encoded in the genes, and so every cell does not make every protein encoded by its genes. Instead, each different cell has specialized requirements for the proteins that it needs to perform its designated tasks. Just like a carpenter needs different tools for different jobs, a cell needs different proteins for different functions. The requirements for specific proteins depend upon where in the body a cell is located. This demand for specific proteins is fulfilled through the selective use of the cell's genetic information.

For example, the cells that make up the eye have specialized tasks to perform so that they can achieve vision. These specialized tasks may require proteins encoded by a certain part of the genetic information that liver cells, which perform different functions, do not need. Since only some of the proteins encoded in the genetic information are needed by eye cells (or liver cells), only some of the proteins encoded in the genetic information are made by each of the different cell types. As a result, eye cells will make the proteins they need and will not make the proteins they do not need. The result is a tremendously important difference in the protein content of cells that form different organs or tissues. This difference in protein content allows certain cells to function as eye cells, liver cells, skin cells, muscle cells, and so on. In this way, the different shapes and functions of the body are determined—and allowed—by each organ's very specific use of the genetic information it carries within its cells.

The different requirements that cells have for proteins can also explain the pattern of symptoms that we see in genetic diseases. For example, cells that require a particular protein, say protein A, may not function properly if there is an alteration in the gene that tells a cell how to make protein A. Other cells, however, that do not need protein A may function completely normally. Consider Duchenne muscular dystrophy (DMD). In DMD, there is an alteration in a protein necessary for proper muscle structure and function. Muscle cells, which require this protein, cannot work well if the protein is not made properly. Therefore, the primary symptoms of DMD are contained within muscular organs and tissues. The most debilitating effects of DMD result from this impairment of muscle function and show up as difficulties in walking and breathing.

When doctors and scientists understand how and where in the body a gene is used and what the protein encoded by the gene does, they can begin to understand the causes of a genetic disease and deduce the reason for the symptoms seen in patients. In addition, scientists can gain insight into better ways to intervene. Genetic research in humans and in other organisms has already demonstrated its ability to provide doctors with insight into the causes of disease. And continued research will be vital to our gaining the ability to detect, properly diagnose, and ultimately treat many human illnesses.

Scientists are also beginning to discover how cells decide which genes to use and which genes to leave alone. Through genetic research, a number of proteins have been identified that control the specific use of genes by cells. But many mysteries remain about how cells promote the use of specific genes and how they control the timing of gene usage throughout life. Future research will undoubtedly help solve these mysteries.

CHAPTER TWO

Chromosomes

As discussed in the previous chapter, the genetic material of human cells is contained on structures called chromosomes. The chromosomes are housed in a region of the cell called the "nucleus." The nucleus is a membrane-bound compartment found inside the cells of all higher organisms, including plants, animals, and humans. It is the room inside the cell that holds the genetic library. The nucleus compartment also contains many elements in addition to the chromosomes. These elements are very important to cellular function and include the proteins that copy the chromosomes before mitosis and read the instructions contained in genes.

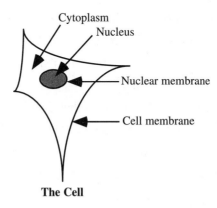

The Cell

FIGURE 2.1   A cell. Cells are the tiny building blocks of the body. Cells are fluid- and protein-filled objects bound by a cell membrane. The inside of a cell is called the "cytoplasm." Within the cytoplasm of cells is a membrane-bound compartment called the nucleus. The nucleus contains the chromosomes.

The chromosomes can be thought of as a sort of scaffolding that holds the genes, the bookshelves that hold the books of the cellular library.

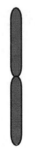

FIGURE 2.2   A chromosome. Human cells have forty-six chromosomes.

The individual genes are spread out along the length of the chromosomes like books would be on a bookshelf. Just like books in a real library, some genes are larger than others and take up more space on the chromosomes than smaller genes. But unlike a well organized library, not all genes on a chromosome necessarily face the same direction.

Besides the genes, chromosomes also contain important structural elements. These structural features are responsible for duplicating the chromosomes completely before mitosis and making certain that exactly one copy of each chromosome gets sorted to each of the newly forming daughter cells during mitosis. These elements ensure that all future cells contain the entire content of the genetic library.

We learned in the last chapter that every cell carries a complete set of genetic information. This is important because cells must have all the reference materials they need to produce all the proteins required for proper function, wherever they are in the body. It is also important that cells carry a complete set of genetic information, so that a complete genetic library can be passed on to the next generation through the sperm and egg.

If cells lack a part of the genetic information, as in the case of many genetic diseases, there is a much greater risk of anomalies in cellular function. For example, think of the genetic material as a cellular library. A cell with a complete library needs only to decide how to use the information. However, a cell with an incomplete library may lack some crucial information. Cells missing genetic information are often unable to perform certain functions. If the information is missing in one generation, it will be missing in the next generation, too.

Consider mitosis. As we learned in the last chapter, cells copy all their chromosomes before dividing and transmit one complete copy to each daughter cell. The alternative to this would be to parcel out the genetic material. If cells had to divide the genetic material into parcels during mitosis and deliver some but not all parcels to individual daughter cells, the dividing cell would have to precisely divide the genetic material and carefully distribute the material to daughter cells. Proper distribution would depend upon a cell knowing the future purpose of each daughter cell so that daughter cells would receive all the information they need. Once a daughter cell was formed with certain genetic material missing, there would be no going back. That cell's capabilities would be permanently limited.

Next, consider the human genetic material—forty-six different chromosomes comprising roughly two meters in length of genetic material. Consider the hundreds of different cell types in the body, each with its own specific function. It is not hard to imagine what a complicated process it could become to parcel out the DNA correctly, so cells do not try. Instead, what cells do is just duplicate and transmit all the genetic information to each new daughter cell. Then cells only need to decide how to use the information.

In humans, the usual chromosome complement of a cell is forty-six chromosomes. These forty-six chromosomes are arranged in twenty-three pairs of like chromosomes. For example, there are two chromosome number 1s, two number 2s, two number 3s, and so on, up to pair 22. The twenty-third chromosome pair consists of the sex chromosomes, the X and the Y chromosomes. Normal human females carry two X chromosomes and normal human males carry one X and one Y chromosome.

In the laboratory, the chromosomes are arbitrarily labeled according to their length and content with chromosome number 1 being the longest. Each chromosome pair carries a specific, constant set of genes. The entire

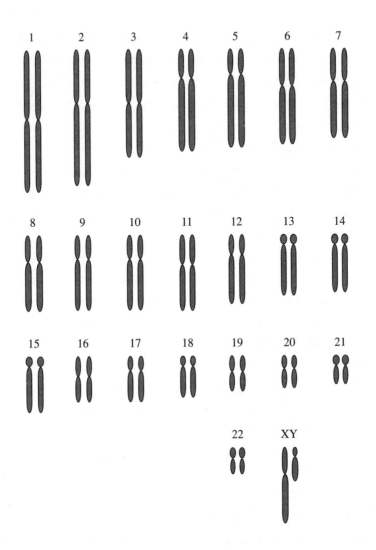

FIGURE 2.3 Diagram showing the chromosome content of a single human cell, forty-six chromosomes in twenty-three pairs. The chromosome number is shown above each pair. Note the relative size differences of the different chromosomes. This diagram is representative of a normal male. Notice the presence of one X and one Y chromosome.

complement of human chromosomes and the genes they contain is called the "human genome."

One member of each of the twenty-three chromosome pairs is inherited from each parent at the time of fertilization. The sperm from the father carries one of each of the twenty-three different chromosomes—one chromosome 1, one chromosome 2, one chromosome 3, and so on. So does the egg from the mother. As a result, half of the chromosomes of a child come from the father and half come from the mother. Fertilization of the egg reconstitutes the total chromosome number to forty-six chromosomes, in twenty-three pairs of chromosomes.

Another way to think about the inheritance of chromosomes is to visualize the chromosomes as forty-six little pieces of string. In each of your cells, imagine that twenty-three of those pieces of string are blue (the ones from your father) and twenty-three of those pieces of string are pink (the ones from your mother). For each different pair of chromosomes, every cell should have one pink and one blue chromosome—i.e., one pink chromosome 1 and one blue chromosome 1, one pink chromosome 2 and one blue chromosome 2, one pink chromosome 3 and one blue chromosome 3, and so on.

By way of example, let us examine the sex chromosomes and learn how sex is determined at conception. Females carry two X chromosomes. As such, a mother can only contribute an egg with an X chromosome to a child. Males carry one X chromosome and one Y chromosome. So the father will make some sperm that carry an X chromosome and some sperm that carry a Y chromosome. Depending on which type of sperm fertilizes the egg, the child will be either a boy or a girl. If the sperm that fertilizes the egg carries an X chromosome, the child will have two X chromosomes, one from each parent, and will be a girl. If the sperm that fertilizes the egg carries a Y chromosome, the child will have an X chromosome from its mother and a Y chromosome from its father, and will be a boy.

It is interesting that, historically speaking, women have been charged by society—or perhaps more precisely by their husbands—with the responsibility of producing male heirs. Some women have even met their deaths at the hands of disgruntled fathers who wanted a son. Take for example the fate of Ann Boleyn, beheaded at the hand of her husband, King Henry VIII of England, apparently for no greater sin than failing to bear him a son. Ironically, as we now know, the Y chromosome that makes a child male could only have come from Henry himself!

CHAPTER THREE

DNA

We hear about "DNA" today in many contexts. From fiction and fantasy in the movies, to fact in court cases where DNA is used to identify suspects, to medicine in the doctor's office where DNA is used to diagnose disease. But what is DNA, really?

The letters DNA are actually an abbreviation for a biological molecule. The abbreviation stands for **d**eoxyribo**n**ucleic **a**cid. DNA is the basic chemical component of the genetic material of living things throughout nature, from bacteria to plants to animals to humans. Even some viruses carry DNA as their genetic material. In man, each of the forty-six chromosomes of a human cell is a single, long molecule of DNA. As we have learned, the DNA molecule is one long bookshelf on each row of the cell's genetic library, and these individual shelves hold the books, or genes, that contain the information required by cells in order to produce proteins.

In describing the structure of the DNA molecule, we must leave our analogy of the library for a moment and think of the DNA molecule itself as a ladder. The sides of the ladder can be broken down into individual units called "nucleotides." Nucleotides are the building blocks of DNA. Each side of the incremental steps of the DNA ladder is made up of one nucleotide. The individual nucleotides are chemically bonded together, end to end, to form a long strand of nucleotides. The strand of nucleotides makes the long sides of the ladder. The rungs of the ladder are made up of chemical bonds called "hydrogen bonds." Hydrogen bonds hold the nucleotides on opposite sides of the DNA ladder together. As a result, the complete DNA molecule is really two long nucleotide strands stuck together by hydrogen bonds.

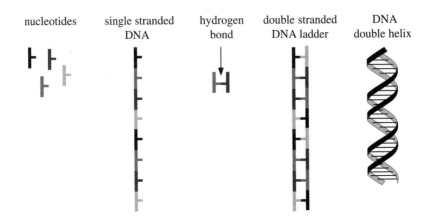

| nucleotides | single stranded DNA | hydrogen bond | double stranded DNA ladder | DNA double helix |

FIGURE 3.1 DNA is made of individual units called nucleotides. Nucleotides combine together in a string to make a single strand of DNA. The single strands of DNA are joined by hydrogen bonds to make the double-stranded DNA ladder. Double-stranded DNA is the form of DNA found in human cells.

The DNA ladder is often referred to as a "double helix." Double because it is a two-sided ladder, and helix because it is twisted in a helix or spiral. Imagine if you were to anchor both sides of the bottom of a ladder to the ground and turn the top in a circle, the resulting spiral would resemble the DNA double helix.

There are four different individual nucleotide building blocks in DNA. The four nucleotides are different because of differences in their chemical structures. They are named adenine, guanine, cytosine, and thymine and are abbreviated A, G, C, and T according to the first letters of their names. Scientists use these abbreviations when talking about nucleotides in DNA.

The four different nucleotides, A, C, G, and T, can each be found on both sides of the DNA ladder. The nucleotides that pair with each other through the hydrogen bonds across the ladder rungs of DNA always associate with each other in the same way. For example, nucleotide A does not pair with nucleotide A, nor with C, nor with G. Instead, nucleotide A always pairs with T. And nucleotide C always pairs with G. A hydrogen-bonded pair of either A-T or C-G is called a "base pair." Each base pair is a step of the DNA ladder, and there are an estimated six billion (6,000,000,000) base pairs in the complete human genome of forty-six chromosomes.

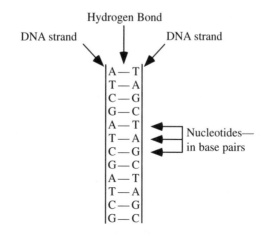

FIGURE 3.2   Diagram showing how the nucleotides pair to form a double-stranded DNA molecule. This drawing shows twelve base pairs of DNA, that is to say it is twelve base pairs long. Notice that there are only two types of base pairs, A-T and C-G. Notice also that each of the different nucleotides can be found on both sides of the DNA ladder.

Because of the precise nature of base pairing, decoding the sequence of one side or strand of the DNA ladder, provides, by inference, the sequence of the other side. Imagine if A always pairs with T. Where you find an A on one nucleotide string, you will always find a T on its mate. As will be described in Chapter 19, this is a useful feature for scientists interested in studying DNA.

The cell also takes advantage of this precise base pairing during mitosis. As we have already learned, the chromosomes are copied or duplicated before cell division so that each new cell contains a complete set of genetic information. When the chromosomes are copied during cell division, the opposite sides of the DNA ladder, or double helix, separate briefly into single strands all along the length of the chromosome. The separation of DNA strands is accomplished by disruption of the hydrogen bonds—somewhat like the unzipping of a zipper. It would be like taking a saw and sawing right down the middle of the DNA ladder, sawing the steps in half. You would be left with two halves of the ladder.

After being separated, the existing sides of the DNA ladder are used as guides or templates for making hydrogen bonds with new nucleotides. The nucleotides pair A to T and C to G, until two DNA molecules appear where one existed before.

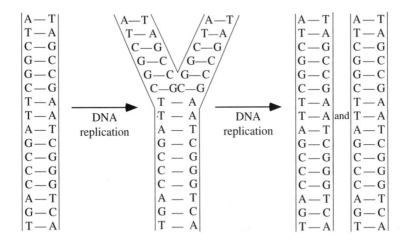

FIGURE 3.3 DNA replication. DNA replication is the process by which cells copy DNA, turning one DNA double helix into two. During replication, the existing DNA molecule is separated into single strands through disruption of its hydrogen bonds. Special proteins in the cell then use the unpaired nucleotides of each existing DNA strand to direct the synthesis of a second, new strand through the formation of new hydrogen bonds.

In each of the two newly formed chromosomes, one side of the DNA ladder is old, from the previous chromosome, and one side is new, from the duplication process. After DNA duplication, also called replication, mitosis can proceed. Remember, during mitosis one copy of each chromosome is allotted to each of the two newly forming daughter cells.

Nucleotides are not only the building blocks of the DNA ladder, but they also serve another, very important purpose. As we will learn in the next two chapters, nucleotides carry the information content, or instructions, of DNA. Basically, nucleotides can be thought of as the alphabet of biology. But instead of having twenty-six letters like the written English alphabet, there are just the four letters in DNA: A, C, G, and T.

The combination of the nucleotide alphabet in a string, much like we string letters together to make words, is how DNA gives a cell instructions. The order of nucleotides in the string is called its "sequence." Just as we put different combinations of letters together to form different words, DNA puts different sequences of nucleotides together to encode different instructions. All the different genes in a cell are simply different sequences of nucleotides that give a cell different sets of instructions for making different proteins. It is this tremendous variety of nucleotide combinations in a DNA sequence that permits all of the different genes for all of the different functions of a cell.

CHAPTER FOUR

Genes and Proteins

So far we have learned that each individual chromosome is a single molecule of DNA and that chromosomes are each made up of long sequences of nucleotides. So are genes.

The very long DNA sequence of each chromosome has mixed within it the shorter DNA sequences that make up individual genes. The genes are said to reside on the chromosomes. Each gene has a specific chromosomal address and, unless something is wrong, each gene is always found in the same place on the same chromosome in all people. In all, there are an estimated 50,000 to 100,000 different genes contained in the genetic information of a human cell—50,000 to 100,000 books in the human genetic library.

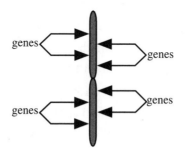

FIGURE 4.1 A chromosome carrying genes all along its length.

We have also already learned that genes provide the cell with the information it needs to function. Much the same way that a computer program provides the information needed to carry out the functions of the machine, our genes provide the information needed for our cells to divide, develop, and function properly.

Functionally, genes are tiny packets of information. Cells use their genes to make proteins. Proteins are the functional interpretation of the genetic information. The proteins perform many different kinds of tasks in cells based on the messages interpreted from the genes.

Some proteins function as structural components of cells and tissues, giving cells their shapes or providing the basis for attachments between cells to hold tissues and organs together. Collagen, an example of a structural protein, is a major component of bone and is also found in skin and cartilage.

Some proteins function as regulatory components that control growth, development, and cell division. Some regulatory proteins make sure that cells divide the right number of times to build an organ or tissue properly. Others help to ensure that the right proteins are available when the cells need them.

Some proteins function as enzymes. Enzymes are proteins that carry out the biochemical reactions within cells to convert one compound to another.

Some proteins function to transport molecules across a cell's membranes. These proteins serve to assort important factors within and among cells.

Finally, some proteins serve to communicate signals or to send messages to and among cells. Hormones are an example of this type of protein.

Some proteins work individually to perform their functions and some work as parts of multi-unit protein complexes. For example, Hemophilia A is a genetic disease caused by alterations in the gene that encodes a protein called "Factor VIII" (factor eight). The Factor VIII protein is found in the blood and helps stop bleeding by assisting in the formation of blood clots. The Factor VIII protein is a single subunit protein that interacts with other, independent proteins to help in blood clot formation. Alterations in the gene can interfere with the ability to make Factor VIII properly. Improperly made Factor VIII can result in symptoms suggestive of an inability to form blood clots such as easy bruising, bleeding into muscles and joints, and longer-than-normal bleeding times from wounds. These symptoms are characteristic of Hemophilia A.

Alternatively, Tay-Sachs disease is caused by alterations in the gene for one of the subunits of a two-subunit enzyme called "Hexosaminidase A," abbreviated "Hex A." The two subunits interact to complete the structure of the Hex A enzyme. In Tay-Sachs disease, alterations in the gene for the α subunit impair the function of the entire Hex A enzyme, even though the β subunit is unaltered. Impairment of the function of the Hex A enzyme interferes with a cell's ability to catalyze an important enzymatic reaction. The symptoms of Tay-Sachs result from the accumulation of the compounds usually degraded by the Hex A enzyme. The impairment of Hex A enzyme function in Tay-Sachs patients causes rapid and progressive loss of neurologic function.

As these examples demonstrate, a cell's protein inventory defines that cell's capabilities. Cells can only perform functions for which they have the necessary proteins to do the jobs. If a cell needs to complete a particular task but it lacks proteins capable of performing that task, the cell and its tissue or organ—or sometimes the entire body—may experience problems because of the deficiency.

If a cell lacks the proteins needed to perform a particular function because of an alteration in the genetic information, a genetic disease is the result. If the function in question is a basic function—one needed by many cells—the resulting genetic condition may be incompatible with life beyond a certain stage of development or growth. Alternatively, if the function is needed only by certain cells at a certain time of life, the clinical effect in the person will depend on the gene defect and the function of the encoded protein.

The DNA sequences that encode genes make up only a small percentage of the entire human genomic DNA sequence. There are many more regions of the genetic content that do not make proteins. Scientists suspect that some of the non-gene DNA plays a role in the structure of the chromosomes and in the maintenance, duplication, and transmission of the chromosomes in their proper form.

In addition, there is quite a bit of DNA in human cells that we know very little about. These mysterious sequences of DNA are interspersed among the genes and the structural elements. They are lengths of DNA that apparently do not code for proteins or serve any other known purpose. Much of this DNA is sometimes called junk DNA or satellite DNA. As will be discussed in Chapter 17, the nucleotide sequence of this DNA can be very different when DNA samples from two different people are compared. The variations that occur in these regions of DNA are often used by scientists to help distinguish between a DNA sample that was taken from one person and one that was taken from another person. This is the basis of forensic applications of DNA testing, such as comparing DNA samples collected at a crime scene from those taken from potential suspects.

CHAPTER FIVE

How Genes Make Proteins

You may have already read somewhere before, perhaps in biology class, the statement, "DNA makes RNA makes protein." While this may sound confusing, complicated, and even intimidating, it is nothing more than a step-by-step description of how cells make proteins.

It is important for cells to make proteins in order to perform their designated tasks. It is also important for cells to maintain their DNA because proteins do not last forever. The life span of many proteins is tightly regulated by cells. As a result, some proteins must be remade periodically if a cell is to continue to function. Also, at different times during its life, a cell may need to make different sets of proteins for doing different jobs. This relentless demand for proteins makes maintenance of the DNA's instructions crucial for cell survival.

The process of "DNA makes RNA makes protein" allows cells to preserve DNA as an unlimited source of information. By acting through the RNA intermediate, DNA is kept intact to be used repeatedly for making the proteins needed throughout the life of a cell.

To make understanding the process simpler, we can break it down into two parts. The first part of the process is where DNA makes RNA. This process is called "transcription." During transcription, DNA is simply copied into RNA.

Transcription

Just like DNA, RNA is an abbreviation. RNA stands for ribonucleic acid. The RNA is made from DNA inside the nucleus of the cell, where the DNA resides. The RNA molecule is made using the double-stranded DNA as a guide or template, and the RNA molecule is a copy of one of the strands of the double-stranded DNA—a copy of one half of the DNA ladder.

The copying of DNA into RNA during transcription requires that the DNA double helix separate briefly, just as it does during replication of the DNA prior to cell division. However, instead of copying the DNA to DNA as in replication, in transcription DNA is copied into RNA. The sequence of the RNA is dictated by the sequence of the DNA.

The order of nucleotides incorporated into the RNA is decided by base pairing with the DNA nucleotides. The purpose of the base pairing between DNA and RNA is to assure that the RNA that gets made is an accurate representation of the nucleotide sequence in the DNA instructions. The base pairing that occurs between RNA and DNA is similar to that between DNA and DNA, where C pairs with G. But RNA contains no T nucleotide. In RNA, the A from DNA pairs with a U. U stands for uridine, the fourth nucleotide in RNA. Uridine is found only in RNA. It is not found in DNA.

The base pairing between DNA and RNA nucleotides is temporary and results in an RNA copy of the DNA strand. After the RNA is made, it separates from the DNA template, and the DNA ladder reforms its double-stranded structure.

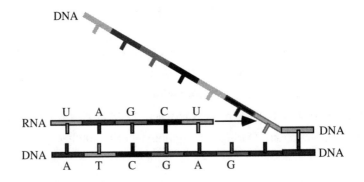

FIGURE 5.1 Transcription. Transcription is the process by which DNA is used as a template to make RNA. The nucleotide sequence of the RNA molecule is dictated by hydrogen bonding of RNA nucleotides to the DNA template. Thus, the RNA is an exact copy of the DNA in a gene.

When a gene is copied into RNA, it is said to be "expressed."

RNA nucleotides are also chemically a little different from DNA nucleotides. RNA is single-stranded instead of double-stranded, so there is not a regular helical ladder structure to RNA. RNA represents a temporary form of the information contained in a gene.

Specific DNA sequences embedded within the gene help in the transcription of the DNA into RNA. At the beginning of a gene, there is a sequence called a "promoter." The promoter prompts the location, timing, and rate of transcription. The promoter helps a cell begin to convert the DNA into RNA.

After the promoter, there are genetic sequences necessary for providing instructions on how to make the protein that the gene is in charge of making. These sequences form the centerpiece of the information of DNA and are called "exons." Exons are the chapters, sentences, and words in the gene books. Without them, a cell would have no instructions for synthesis of actual proteins.

Mixed in with these instructional sequences are sequences that will eventually be removed from the RNA before a protein is made. These sequences, called "intervening sequences" or "introns," are of unknown function, but they occur in all higher organisms such as plants, animals, and humans.

At the end of a gene, there are DNA sequences involved in stopping transcription. These sequences function in an opposite role to the promoter.

After transcription, the RNA is modified to remove the introns, the sequences that will not be used to encode the protein. These and other modifications prepare the RNA for export from the nucleus. Once modified, the RNA travels from the nucleus to the cytoplasm.

The cytoplasm is the area of the cell outside the nucleus but still within the cell membrane. Once outside the nucleus in the cytoplasm, the RNA guides the production of proteins through the second part of the process, called "translation."

Translation

Translation is how RNA makes protein. Translation is based on the instructions set forth in the RNA. It is carried out on cellular structures

The Structure of a Gene

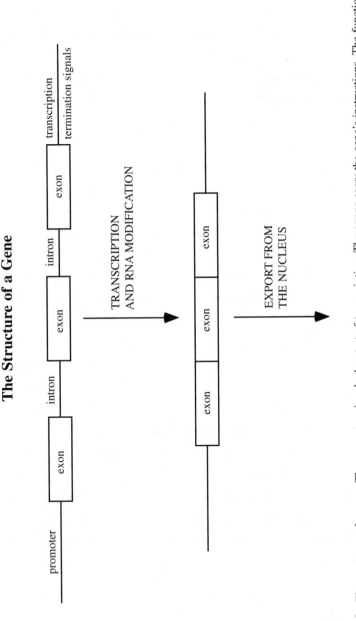

FIGURE 5.2 The structure of a gene. The promoter signals the start of transcription. The exons carry the gene's instructions. The function of the introns is unknown. The transcription termination signals tell the proteins that accomplish transcription where and how to stop.

called "ribosomes." Ribosomes are the translators, the machines on which the genetic message of RNA is read and converted, or translated, into functional proteins.

Proteins are composed of chemical components called amino acids. Like the nucleotides of DNA, amino acids are the individual building blocks of proteins. And just like nucleotides, amino acids are combined end to end in a string to make a protein.

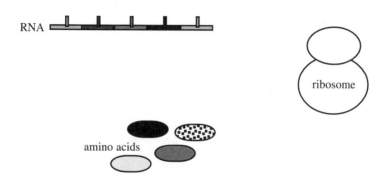

FIGURE 5.3   The components of translation. Ribosomes are the cell's protein-making machines. They bring RNA together with amino acids.

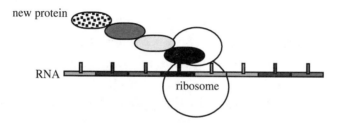

FIGURE 5.4   The process of translation. The ribosomes bring RNA and amino acids into close contact. The RNA is used as a guide to determine the order in which the different amino acids are incorporated into a newly forming protein.

The completion of translation results in a protein, built specifically as described by the original gene and its RNA intermediary. But how is the nucleotide message of a gene converted to amino acids? What is the secret code?

First, it is important to know that there are twenty different amino acids in cells, twenty different building blocks with which proteins can be made. The order in which the amino acids are linked together to form a protein is dictated by the RNA sequence as programmed by the gene.

But instead of a one-to-one relationship, like the copying of DNA nucleotides into RNA nucleotides, every three nucleotides in RNA encode just one amino acid. Because of this three-to-one relationship, the protein coding portion of an RNA molecule has three times as many nucleotides as the resulting protein has amino acids. The three-nucleotide groups in RNA that specify a single amino acid in a protein are called "codons."

| 30 nucleotides |

RNA codons: CGU   CAU   CAA   UCU UAU   CCG GGU CUU GCG   GGA
protein amino acids: arginine-histidine-glutamine-serine-tyrosine-proline-glycine-leucine-alanine-glycine

| 10 amino acids |

FIGURE 5.5 The number of nucleotides in the protein-coding region of an RNA strand are in a three-to-one ratio with the number of amino acids in the encoded protein. Three nucleotides in an RNA make one codon. Each codon specifies one amino acid.

The codons can be thought of as the words in the genetic language of DNA. Different three-nucleotide words make different codons. Different codons signify different amino acids. So when different codons are linked together in the sequence of an RNA, different amino acid sequences are incorporated into the protein. The ribosomes are the machines that recognize the codons and translate the message in RNA into amino acids for proteins.

Taken together, the DNA nucleotide sequence, through the order of the nucleotides in RNA, is how DNA programs RNA. The RNA nucleotide sequence, through codons, is how RNA programs proteins. This is the

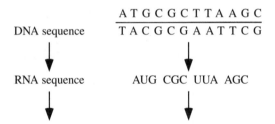

DNA sequence
A T G C G C T T A A G C
T A C G C G A A T T C G

RNA sequence   AUG CGC UUA AGC

Amino acid sequence: methionine-arginine-leucine-serine

FIGURE 5.6 A few of the different codons in RNA, which are represented by different three-nucleotide sequences. Note how different nucleotide sequences from DNA, in the form of different RNA codons, specify particular amino acids.

genetic code. And this is how, because of transcription and translation, DNA makes RNA makes protein.

Differences in DNA nucleotide sequence among genes is how a cell makes so many different RNAs during transcription. Different RNAs is how a cell makes so many different proteins during translation. Different proteins make a variety of cellular functions possible.

CHAPTER SIX

Mutations and Other Alterations in DNA

So far, we have learned that the sequence of nucleotides in genes specifies the sequence of amino acids in proteins, and that DNA uses an intermediary, RNA, to convey its message to the protein-assembly machines called ribosomes. We have also learned that cells can only perform functions for which they have the proteins to do the job. Genetic disease is the result when improper messages stored in the DNA cause certain necessary protein functions to be missing or altered.

Improper messages in the DNA are the result of variations in the nucleotide sequences of genes. These variations appear as DNA sequences that have been changed from sequences usually found in lots of individuals, to sequences seen only in individuals with certain medical symptoms. These medically significant variations in DNA sequence are often called "mutations."

Mutations in DNA can be caused either by errors that occur during DNA duplication, by agents that damage or break DNA, or by errors during a process called "recombination," which is discussed in more detail in Chapter 9.

Errors during DNA duplication can occur if there are problems in copying the DNA. No matter how hard a cell tries, no process is perfect, and errors can come from improperly functioning proteins or from failure to correct random mistakes. For example, if the proteins responsible for duplicating the DNA do not work properly, they can cause errors in the new DNA sequence as it is copied from the template.

Suppose one of the proteins responsible for duplicating DNA is malfunctioning because it carries a mutation of its own. Such a protein might make errors more frequently than usual when duplicating the DNA. Under these circumstances, cells can become error prone. If these proteins do not replicate the DNA accurately, the errors can be incorporated into the newly forming DNA strand.

On the other hand, sometimes mistakes in replicating DNA just happen, as if by accident. Because maintaining the DNA is so important, cells have a built-in system to proofread DNA and detect and correct errors. However, if this proofreading system fails to correct any errors that might have occurred during DNA duplication, then permanent changes can occur in the DNA sequence of a cell.

Mutations in DNA can also be caused by DNA damage from either internal agents such as harmful or damaging metabolic products or external agents such as chemicals, toxins, or radiation. Such agents can damage nucleotides singly or in groups, or in some cases even break the DNA ladder.

Uncorrected errors or DNA damage can be passed to daughter cells during mitosis and, subsequently, to all future daughter cells in future mitoses. If an error occurs in a cell destined to become a sperm or egg, future generations can carry the mutation.

The term "mutation" generally implies a harmful effect on a protein's function as a result of a nucleotide sequence change, but many nucleotide sequence changes occur without causing harm to the functions of proteins. If a nucleotide sequence change is not harmful to a protein, it is not likely to result in genetic disease.

Sequence changes that do not cause genetic disease are often called "polymorphisms" or "base substitutions" instead of mutations. Poly meaning "many," morphisms meaning "forms," polymorphism is used by scientists to describe the variety of different nucleotide sequences that can be found in any particular segment of DNA. Segments of DNA that commonly vary from one person to the next are said to be polymorphic. Using a separate term helps to distinguish the innocuous medical effect of polymorphic changes in DNA sequence from the more harmful mutations that can cause noticeable problems in protein function. Clinically speaking, changes in DNA sequence are only important when they result in some sort of medical impairment that causes them to be noted symptomatically as a genetic disease.

However, polymorphisms that do not cause harmful variations in DNA sequence are also important for several reasons. Polymorphisms make each of us genetically and physically unique. Variations in DNA sequences from person to person allow for different blood types and differences in hair and eye color, height, and weight. Only identical twins share exactly the same DNA.

Identical twins occur when a single embryo splits sometime shortly after fertilization to form two embryos. These two embryos then grow into two separate fetuses and are born as two separate babies. However, since the babies originated from a single fertilized egg, they share exactly the same DNA. Fraternal twins are not genetically identical because they grow from two separate fertilized eggs, each with its own unique genetic content.

Individuality in DNA sequence is also important because it can be used by scientists in the laboratory as a tool for distinguishing between individuals. One way these individual differences in DNA can be useful is in determining paternity. We have already learned that children inherit half of their genes from their mothers and half from their fathers. As such, a child will always share DNA sequences with both his or her father and his or her mother. Comparison of specific DNA sequences in a child with the DNA sequences of an alleged father can often help determine whether or not the alleged father did in fact make a genetic contribution to the child. For example, if the alleged father and child share matching DNA sequences at a number of highly polymorphic genetic sites, then the likelihood that the man made a genetic contribution to the child becomes more likely with each identical DNA sequence identified. If, however, there are a number of DNA sequences in the child that differ from those carried by the alleged father, then it is unlikely that the alleged father could have contributed those sequences to the child, and paternity can be called into question.

Comparison of DNA polymorphisms between individuals is also frequently used to determine if a DNA sample obtained from an identified person is the same as that obtained from an unidentified source. For example, DNA sequence comparison can be used in criminal investigations in which DNA samples taken from crime scenes are compared with DNA samples from one or a few suspects. If the DNA is found to be identical, then it may be considered as evidence that supports a particular person being at a particular place. Another potential use for this technology is to identify bodily remains, such as in wartime or in cases of crimes against unknown victims. The varied applications of DNA testing for the identification of individuals and paternity testing is discussed in more detail in Chapter 17.

DNA polymorphisms can occur throughout the genome. Many polymorphisms in DNA sequence will occur in chromosomal regions that do not contain genes, thereby not affecting any protein. For example, if a segment of a chromosome is changed but that segment does not constitute part of a gene, clearly there will be no effect on a protein. Since these changes are not likely to result in a change in a protein, they are not likely to be detected outside a research environment because there will be no physical effect resulting from the sequence change.

Sometimes, however, changes in DNA sequence occur within genes. When this happens, it is important to consider whether the DNA sequence change affects the sequence of a protein. Changes in DNA sequence do not always alter the sequence of the protein. This is possible because the genetic code is redundant.

Imagine for a moment that with four different nucleotides and three nucleotides in a row determining a codon, there are 4 x 4 x 4 = 64 possible different three-nucleotide codons for specifying the amino acids to be added to a protein.

As we learned in the last chapter, there are not sixty-four different amino acids—only twenty. What this means is that several different three-nucleotide codons can represent the same amino acid. For example, the codons C-G-A, C-G-C, C-G-G, and C-G-U all specify the addition of the same amino acid to a protein—the amino acid arginine. As a result, the genetic code is called "redundant," meaning that several different codons may direct the addition of the same amino acid to a protein.

Because of the redundancy of the genetic code, some changes in DNA sequence may alter the nucleotide sequence of a gene and its RNA, but not the amino acid sequence of a protein. This can occur if the new codon still

```
AAA CAA GAA UAA
AAC CAC GAC UAC
AAG CAG GAG UAG
AAU CAU GAU UAU

ACA CCA GCA UCA
ACC CCC GCC UCC
ACG CCG GCG UCG
ACU CCU GCU UCU

AGA CGA GGA UGA
AGC CGC GGC UGC
AGG CGG GGG UGG
AGU CGU GGU UGU

AUA CUA GUA UUA
AUC CUC GUC UUC
AUG CUG GUG UUG
AUU CUU GUU UUU
```

FIGURE 6.1   All sixty-four possible codons are shown as different groups of three nucleotides.

Codon	Amino Acid
GCA GCC GCG GCU	ALANINE
CUA CUC CUG CUU	LEUCINE
AAC AAU	ASPARAGINE
AAA AAG	LYSINE

FIGURE 6.2   Redundancy of genetic code for just four of the twenty amino acids. Note that several different codons can signal the same amino acid.

specifies the same amino acid. Notice in Figure 6.2 how a change of codon from GCA to GCC in the RNA still specifies the amino acid alanine. If this change were to happen in a real gene, the protein encoded would probably be unchanged. Such changes that do not alter the protein's sequence should not affect the protein's function. Because this type of DNA change is unlikely to result in a measurable deficiency in the functioning of a protein, it is unlikely to cause a physical effect on a person. Medically speaking, such changes are considered to be fairly insignificant and would probably not be detected without genetic research.

Alternatively, some changes in DNA sequences do result in changes in a protein. For example, if a change in DNA sequence results in a codon that calls for a different amino acid, there is likely to be a change in the encoded protein's sequence. Sometimes these amino acid changes will not have a recognized effect on the functioning of a protein. Such changes are unlikely to be detected outside a research environment, but they are interesting to note.

Keep in mind, however, that not all amino acid changes are irrelevant. Sometimes amino acid changes will negatively affect the functioning of the protein, but only under certain circumstances. Such mild mutations are usually well tolerated by the protein and by the individual, and may show an effect on growth, development, or health only in extreme environmental conditions. Since protein function is not greatly affected by these alterations except in extreme circumstances and the carriers of these changes rarely suffer symptoms, it is impossible to know exactly how many such changes occur in human genes.

A clinical example of a mutation in a protein that is often observed only under certain environmental conditions is glucose 6-phosphate dehydrogenase (G6PD) deficiency. G6PD deficiency is the most common enzyme deficiency in humans, and it can result in severe hemolytic anemia. Some carriers of mutations in this gene suffer mild to moderate chronic anemia. However, more frequently, carriers of G6PD mutations are generally healthy and only show symptoms of severe hemolytic anemia when they take a certain anti-malaria drug or certain antibiotics, or when they ingest fava beans.

In contrast, mutations that alter the sequence of a gene in a way that is inconsistent with proper functioning of the protein will result in a protein deficiency. This type of mutation may cause genetic disease if the protein is crucial to a particular cellular function. Hemophilia A, as described in Chapter 4, is an example of a genetic disease caused by mutations that affect a protein's function.

Finally, some changes in DNA sequence can impair the proper transcription or processing of RNA. For example, if a change in DNA sequence prevents transcription or inhibits the removal of an intron, a protein may not get made properly.

Several types of mutations are known to occur. "Deletion mutations" are mutations where part of a gene is lost or missing. In a deletion mutation, a segment of the DNA sequence of a gene has been removed. Deletions can occur at any point in a chromosome or gene—the beginning, the middle, or the end. The amount of the genetic material missing and its location are often critical to whether the remainder of the gene can produce a functional protein. Cystic fibrosis (CF) and Duchenne muscular dystrophy (DMD) are both genetic diseases in which deletion mutations within the gene responsible for the disease are a common cause.

"Duplication mutations" are mutations in which a gene or part of a gene appears more times than it normally would. Duplications can be very small, just a few nucleotides long, or very large, covering a sizable length of DNA sequence. Duplications can increase the length of a gene because of the presence of additional gene sequences and can have a devastating impact on the functioning of the encoded protein. Duplications involving whole genes can result in too many copies of a gene within a cell. If there are too many copies of a gene, more protein than usual may be made. If too much of a particular protein disturbs a cell's normal functioning, then the duplication mutation can cause medical symptoms. Charcot-Marie-Tooth disease Type 1A is caused by a duplication mutation.

"Insertion mutations" are mutations in which additional material is present that is not normally in the gene. In an insertion mutation, the new material can come from some other place in the cell's genetic material or from some external source of genetic material such as a virus. Most viruses do not insert their genetic material into that of a cell, but retroviruses such as HIV do. This means that the viral sequence, once inserted into the DNA, will be present in that cell for the rest of its life and in all of its daughter cells. The size and location of the additional DNA within the gene are critical to its impact on the expression and function of the gene and the protein it produces.

"Inversion mutations" are mutations where a segment of a gene is flipped around backwards. In an inversion mutation, the front end of a sequence of DNA becomes the tail end. Inversion mutations in genes can alter the amino acid sequence of all or part of a protein. Hemophilia A is an example of a genetic disease that can sometimes be caused by an inversion mutation.

Sometimes the term "rearrangement mutation" is used. Broadly defined, the term rearrangement describes mutations that scramble the sequence of a gene. The term rearrangement mutation is often used to describe inversion mutations. Rearrangements of any type in the nucleotide sequence of a gene can be problematic because they scramble the genetic information and prevent proteins from being assembled properly.

Deletion, duplication, insertion, and rearrangement mutations can occur during DNA replication or as a result of DNA damage when a DNA molecule is broken and rejoined improperly, causing a disruption of the normal nucleotide sequence.

A "point mutation" is a type of mutation in which a single nucleotide substitution occurs within a segment of DNA. Point mutations exchange one nucleotide for another. They are most often caused by DNA damage from harmful substances or by errors during DNA replication. However, since the genetic code is redundant and amino acids can be encoded by more than one codon, a point mutation does not necessarily change the amino acid incorporated into a protein. Point mutations that alter the amino acid sequence of the protein are obviously more likely to impair a protein's function than those that do not alter the amino acid sequence of a protein.

β-thalassemia is an example of a genetic disease that is commonly caused by point mutations. β-thalassemia was first described in individuals of Mediterranean descent, but can also be observed in other populations. In β-thalassemia, point mutations occur in the β-globin gene. The β-globin gene encodes a critical component of hemoglobin, the molecule in red blood cells that carries oxygen throughout the body. In β-thalassemia, point mutations in the β-globin gene result in a failure of cells to make a proper hemoglobin molecule. Failure to produce hemoglobin properly can impair a red blood cell's ability to carry oxygen. Point mutations in the β-globin gene can result in symptoms such as anemia and growth failure.

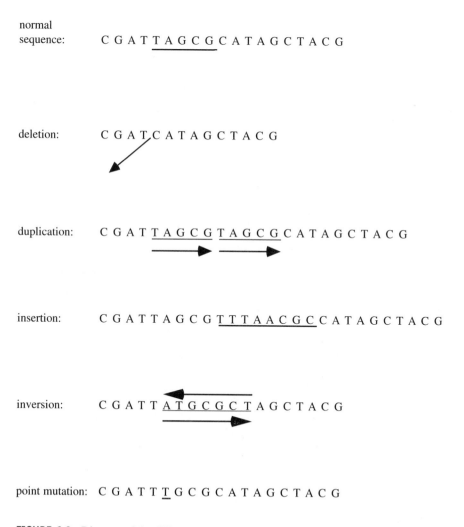

FIGURE 6.3 Diagram of the different kinds of gene mutations.

CHAPTER SEVEN

How Mutations Affect
Genes and Proteins

Mutations in genes can have a variety of effects on proteins. In the previous chapter, we learned that mutations occurring within the part of a gene that specifies the amino acid sequence of a protein can affect how that protein works. These types of mutations, which affect a protein's function, can be classified by the type of change they cause. For example, mutations that result in a protein that can no longer perform its intended function are called "loss of function mutations."

Loss of function mutations can result in physical or medical problems because a crucial job within a cell is not getting done. For example, a fairly common genetic disorder called phenylketonuria (PKU) occurs when a mutation affecting an enzyme called phenylalanine hydroxylase results in the inability of that enzyme to convert phenylalanine to tyrosine. This loss of enzyme activity causes the buildup of phenylalanine in cells. PKU can be extremely debilitating and may result in severe mental retardation if not treated early or if patients do not follow the prescribed treatment plan. PKU is effectively treated by dietary restriction to reduce and control the ingestion of phenylalanine.

Mutations that affect the performance of both the mutant and normal copies of a gene can also be particularly devastating. This type of mutation is called a "dominant negative mutation." In dominant negative mutations, the protein made by the mutant copy of a gene interferes with the protein made by the normal copy of the gene.

Osteogenesis imperfecta (OI) is an example of a dominant negative mutation. In OI, mutations occur in genes that encode a form of collagen. Collagen is used by our bodies to make bones and certain other tissues.

43

Collagen exists in our bodies as a multi-unit complex made up of three collagen molecules. OI occurs when a mutation in one of the collagen genes interferes with the body's ability to make normal collagen complexes. The characteristic symptoms of OI include bone deformations, bone fragility, hearing loss, and abnormalities in tooth development. Some types of OI are mild while others can be lethal.

Typically, in dominant negative mutations, the patient is better off, clinically speaking, with a complete absence of a gene than with a mutated gene. This is because a reduced amount of protein, if it is normal, may have a less severe medical effect than the presence of a malfunctioning protein that damages the assembly of an entire complex. For example, in OI, the absence of a collagen gene is sometimes less severe medically than the presence of a collagen gene with a mutation in it. In other words, less collagen may be better if it is normal collagen than a normal amount of collagen that is improperly formed.

Mutations that change the sequence of a protein and cause proteins to acquire a function they did not previously possess—"gain of function mutations"—can result in physical effects due to the gain of function if the new function is harmful to cells. For example, it is thought that the altered protein involved in Huntington disease carries some new, as yet unknown function, and that this gain of function causes the symptoms of the disease.

As noted in the previous chapter, not all mutations occur within the coding portion of a gene. Genes have other important functional elements that are subject to variations in DNA sequence. For example, mutations can occur within the leader sequence of a gene called the promoter, described in Chapter 5. Promoter mutations are likely to affect the amount of RNA produced from a gene. Mutations that affect the rate or amount of transcription of a gene can alter the amount of a protein produced in cells. If an optimal amount of protein is required for normal functioning, changing the level either up or down can cause problems.

For example, in β-thalassemia, mutations in the promoter region of the β-globin gene reduce the amount of RNA that gets made. Too little β-globin RNA results in too little hemoglobin in red blood cells. The reduced amount of hemoglobin impairs the ability of red blood cells to carry oxygen. Red blood cells that do not carry enough oxygen can cause anemia, changes in bone structure, and growth failure—all of which are symptoms of β–thalassemia.

Mutations in genes may also affect the proper removal of introns from an RNA during the RNA processing that occurs after transcription. Such mutations can affect the level of normal RNA produced from a gene. These types of mutations are called "splice site mutations" or "splicing mutations" because they affect the way the different parts of RNA are spliced together during post-transcriptional processing. Splice site mutations can alter the sequence of the protein made because of the improper removal of necessary sequences from an RNA molecule or the improper retention of intron sequences within an RNA molecule. β–thalassemia can also be caused by this type of mutation.

DNA mutations can occur in any kind of gene. Mutations can occur in genes for structural proteins or regulatory proteins or enzymes. If a mutation occurs in a structural protein, the medical effects are likely to be on the assembly and structure of organs, tissues, or the body as a whole. Depending upon where the protein is needed, certain organs such as the heart or bones may not form properly.

For example, in OI, collagen is an important structural protein of bone. Mutations in collagen genes alter the assembly and structure of bones, and this defect is reflected in the characteristic skeletal symptoms of the disease. With other types of congenital defects such as congenital heart defects, it will be important for scientists to characterize the genes that are important for properly building a heart. Knowing the genes involved can help us learn about how a heart is constructed and how to fix one that was not built properly. Many genes relating to heart development have already been found, but many more certainly remain to be identified.

Mutations in regulatory proteins can affect the timing of production of crucial proteins or the timing of cell divisions and cell maturity. Such mutations may alter the structure, development, or function of organs and tissues, or the timing of changes in the body during development. Mutations in genes that regulate the rate of cell division have been found to be responsible for some types of cancer. As will be discussed in more detail in

Chapter 12, cancer is a disease of uncontrolled cell division caused by the disrupted regulation of the number of times and rate at which cells divide. Disruption of cell division can result in constantly dividing cells that invade and disturb tissues, causing tumors.

Mutations in enzymes can alter the biochemical processes of the body and its organs, tissues, and cells. Remember, enzymes are proteins that are responsible for converting certain substances in the body into other substances. Defects in enzymes can result in deficiencies of necessary components or buildup of inappropriate compounds. PKU, as described earlier in this chapter, is an example of an enzymatic disorder.

Mutations in genes are passed from parent to child when the chromosome that carries the mutated gene is passed from parent to child. When this occurs, the risk for the disease is also passed from parent to child. However, if a parent does not pass the chromosome carrying the mutated gene to a child, then the child will not be at increased risk for developing or transmitting the disease.

But just inheriting a mutation in a gene is not always enough to result in a genetic disease. The risk of a child developing a particular genetic disease also depends upon the type of mutation that has been inherited and the effect the mutation has on cellular function. This process of transmitting mutations and genetic diseases from one generation to the next is described in more detail in the next three chapters.

CHAPTER EIGHT

Passing Genes to the Next Generation

Genes are passed from one generation to the next on chromosomes. Chromosomes are passed from one generation to the next through the germ cells—sperm and eggs. When sperm and egg cells are made, they get their chromosomes from the parent who makes them. We learned in Chapter 2 that normal human cells contain forty-six chromosomes, but human sperm and egg cells each contain twenty-three chromosomes—one of each of the different chromosomes. So if a human cell contains forty-six chromosomes in twenty-three pairs, how are these sperm and egg cells with only twenty-three chromosomes—and no pairs—made?

Sperm and egg cells are produced by a unique cellular process, called "meiosis." Meiosis is designed specifically to reduce the numbers of chromosomes carried in a sperm or egg from forty-six to twenty-three—reducing the number from two of each chromosome to one of each chromosome.

Meiosis occurs only in cells destined to become sperm or eggs. Meiosis begins much like mitosis does. Initially, the genetic material in the cell is duplicated. But instead of a single cell division, as in mitosis, two cell divisions follow the duplication of the genetic material in meiosis.

During the first cell division of meiosis, the twenty-three pairs of duplicated chromosomes are separated so that each daughter cell receives only one of each of the twenty-three different chromosomes. In this way, a sperm or egg reduces the chromosome count from forty-six duplicated chromosomes in the initial cell to twenty-three duplicated chromosomes in the two daughter cells. Since there is a reduction in chromosome number during the first cell division of meiosis, it is often called a "reduction division."

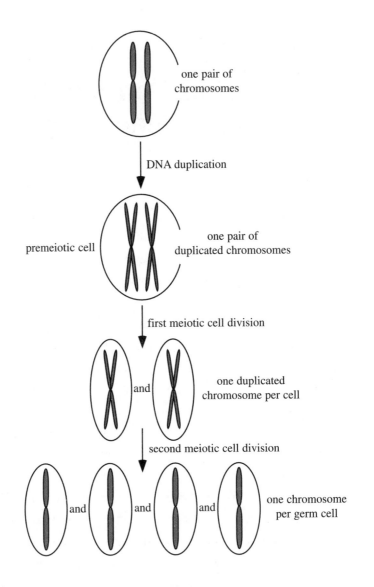

one pair of chromosomes

DNA duplication

premeiotic cell   one pair of duplicated chromosomes

first meiotic cell division

and   one duplicated chromosome per cell

second meiotic cell division

and   and   and   one chromosome per germ cell

FIGURE 8.1   Meiosis, diagrammed in a cell containing only one, paired chromosome. Meiosis is the process by which sperm and egg cells are generated. Note that during the first cell division of meiosis the chromosome pairs are separated such that one member of each pair goes to each daughter cell. During the second cell division, the duplicated chromosomes are split. During meiosis, the chromosome number is reduced from forty-six to twenty-three. This reduction in chromosome number helps to keep the amount of genetic material carried in cells constant from generation to generation.

During the second cell division of meiosis, the duplicated chromosomes are split in two so that each final cell receives one chromosome of each of the twenty-three different chromosomes. It is through the second cell division, a cell division that occurs without DNA duplication, that the final chromosome content of sperm and eggs is achieved. Because of meiosis, the chromosome content of human cells remains constant from generation to generation.

In males, each meiosis results in the formation of four sperm cells. The first cell division results in two cells. In the second cell divisions, these two cells divide to create four cells.

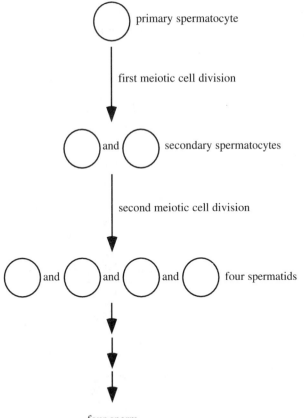

FIGURE 8.2   Male meiosis. Male meiosis results in the production of four sperm.

However, in females, each meiosis results in the formation of only one egg. The first cell division produces one cell that will divide again to become the egg. The second cell that is produced contains little but the separated genetic material. This cell is called a polar body. In the second cell division of female meiosis, which occurs only after fertilization by a sperm, the cell that is to become the egg divides again to create the egg and a second polar body. The polar bodies are eventually lost, while the resulting egg combines its genetic material with that of the sperm, and mitosis ensues.

Since sperm and egg cells carry only one of each of the twenty-three chromosomes, they are said to be "haploid" ("ha" meaning "one" and "ploid" meaning "multiplied by"). Other cells of the body that carry twenty-three pairs

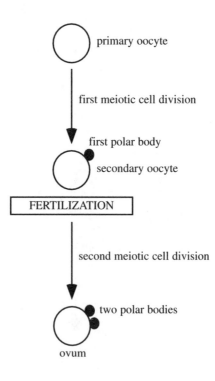

FIGURE 8.3 Female meiosis. Female meiosis results in the production of one egg and two polar bodies.

of chromosomes are said to be "diploid" ("di" meaning "two"). Diploid human cells carry a complete chromosome content of forty-six chromosomes.

Cells that have some variation in the number of chromosomes from the usual twenty-three pairs can sometimes cause genetic disease. Cells that do not carry the appropriate number of chromosomes are said to be "aneuploid" ("an" meaning "not" and "euploid" meaning "exact"). Aneuploid cells, if present in large numbers, can result in a population of cells that do not function properly because of an imbalance in the amount of genetic material and proteins.

Aneuploid cells can appear during meiosis or mitosis when errors occur in chromosome sorting. Errors in chromosome sorting cause an improper number of chromosomes to be distributed to daughter cells. Aneuploidy that occurs during meiosis can seriously impair the viability of a fetus.

Down syndrome is a commonly occurring chromosomal aneuploidy in which cells have an extra, or third, copy of the material that makes chromosome 21. Down syndrome is also sometimes called "trisomy 21"—"trisomy" meaning "three," with "21" referring to chromosome 21. Down syndrome occurs in about one in 800 live births. Commonly noted symptoms of Down syndrome include some variable degree of mental retardation, short stature, and characteristic facial features. Congenital heart defects are also common in babies born with Down syndrome. In the majority of Down syndrome patients, the syndrome is caused by the presence of an extra copy of chromosome 21. In some cases though, extra chromosome 21 material is attached to another chromosome. Studying the origin of the extra chromosome 21 material can help medical professionals determine the likelihood that Down syndrome will recur in future offspring.

Maternal age seems to have an effect in Down syndrome. Mothers over age 30 have a greater per-pregnancy risk of having a Down syndrome baby than do younger mothers. However, this is not to say that younger women cannot have a child with Down syndrome. They can and do. It is the proportion of Down syndrome to non-Down syndrome fetuses that increases with the age of the mother.

Turner syndrome is another commonly seen chromosomal aneuploidy. In Turner syndrome, cells lack a sex chromosome or a major part of one.

Turner syndrome is sometimes called "monosomy X," meaning one of chromosome X. Turner syndrome occurs in about 1 in 5,000 females. Turner syndrome patients often have lower than average height, abnormal development of internal sex organs, and heart defects. In about half of Turner syndrome cases, cells carry a single X chromosome with no Y chromosome or second X chromosome and only forty-five chromosomes in all. However, other types of chromosomal alterations also occur in Turner syndrome and can result in a similar loss of chromosomal material. These other types of genetic alterations are generally fairly complicated, and analysis of the chromosomes from a patient is often required to determine the precise cause of the syndrome.

Some other frequently observed chromosomal aneuploidies include trisomy 13, presence of a third copy of chromosome 13 material; trisomy 18, presence of a third copy of chromosome 18 material; and Klinefelter syndrome, which is caused by the presence of more than one X chromosome in the presence of a Y chromosome. Individuals with Klinefelter syndrome carry two or more X chromosomes together with one Y chromosome, and forty-seven or more chromosomes in all. Trisomy 13 is seen in about one in 15,000 live births. Trisomy 18 is seen in about one in 5,000 live births and Klinefelter syndrome is seen in about one in 1,000 males.

Some carriers of aneuploidies may be "mosaic." In a mosaic individual, some cells carry the usual number of chromosomes while others carry an unusual number. If the cells carrying an unusual number of chromosomes are few, the effect on the individual may be less than for an individual in whom most cells carry the abnormality. Mosaic aneuploidy, therefore, sometimes results in more mildly affected individuals than complete aneuploidy, where every cell is affected.

CHAPTER NINE

Genetic Variation, Independent Assortment, and Recombination

With the exception of identical twins, each of us is genetically and physically unique. We each have, among other things, our own height, weight, hair and eye color, facial characteristics, personalities, likes, and dislikes. Many of these individual characteristics are influenced by our environment and our experiences. For example, if a person lifts weights in the gym, he or she is likely to be more muscular than someone who doesn't.

However, many of our traits are strongly influenced by our genes. One such trait, blood type, is determined by our genes, and we cannot do anything to change it. Some other characteristics, such as cholesterol levels, are more in the middle—influenced by both our genes and our environment. For example, a person may have naturally high cholesterol levels, but that person can lower those levels by the way he or she eats or exercises or by taking medicines.

Variability in DNA is responsible for many of the traits that vary from person to person. Normally, the genes on human chromosomes are all arranged in the same order in all people. But despite all our genes being located in the same places on our chromosomes, the DNA nucleotide sequences are not always the same in all people at every position in the genome. This is most clearly and dramatically illustrated by genetic disease. If we all had exactly the same DNA, we would all have exactly the same disease—or lack thereof.

Blood type is a non-disease-related example of how we can be genetically different from each other. There are several different blood types in man. Some people are O positive, some are O negative. Others are A positive, A negative, B positive, B negative, AB positive, or AB negative. Our genes determine our blood type, and if we all had the same DNA sequences throughout our genomes, we would not have different blood types.

Our individual genetic variability is ensured by a number of factors. First, alterations that occur in nucleotide sequences during DNA replication in mitosis and meiosis or through DNA damage can help to make us unique by changing the sequence of genes in our cells. These changes can be established in the population when they are passed from parent to child and on through later generations.

Second, there are two well-defined processes that occur during meiosis that add to our genetic individuality. One process, called "independent assortment," provides for shuffling of the chromosomes from one generation to the next. The other, called "recombination," provides for shuffling of the genes.

Independent Assortment

As discussed in the previous chapter, in the first cell division of meiosis, one chromosome of each of the twenty-three pairs of chromosomes is distributed to each of the newly forming daughter cells. This gives a sperm or egg the appropriate amount of genetic information—one each of the twenty-three different chromosomes.

Remember that in normal circumstances, a person carries one set of twenty-three chromosomes that is inherited from his or her mother and one set of twenty-three that is inherited from his or her father. But when that person conducts meiosis to make sperm and egg cells, these chromosome sets are not retained intact. As such, sperm and eggs do not necessarily contain the exact same groups of chromosomes that were inherited from the person's parents.

To better illustrate this, let's consider the twenty-three chromosomes you inherited from your mother. This set of chromosomes is not necessarily passed to any of your children as a set, but are mixed with the twenty-three chromosomes that you inherited from your father.

Think back to our example of the forty-six chromosomes in your cells as forty-six little pieces of string, with twenty-three blue from your father and

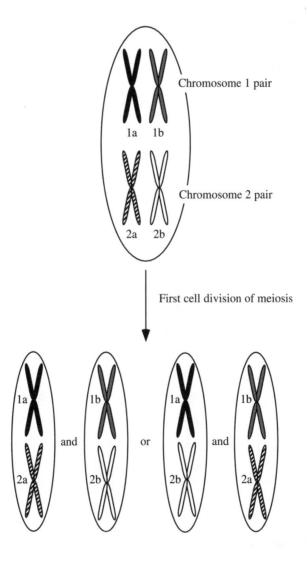

FIGURE 9.1 Diagram showing how independent assortment can occur for two different chromosomes. Notice that, on the left, chromosome 1a sorts with chromosome 2a, and 1b sorts with 2b. Alternatively, on the right, the opposite occurs where chromosome 1a sorts with 2b, and 1b sorts with 2a. The choice of how these chromosomes are assorted during cell division is random.

twenty-three pink from your mother. Without independent assortment, the egg or sperm you make would contain either an all pink or an all blue chromosome set. But this does not happen. When a person makes sperm or eggs, the twenty-three chromosomes contained within those sperm and eggs are a mixture—some are pink and some are blue—but there is still only a single chromosome of each pair.

The choice of which chromosome of any distinct pair goes to a given daughter cell is random for each different chromosome. As a result, the chromosome sets get shuffled from parent to child. Notice in Figure 9.1 how with two chromosomes, there are four possible combinations of chromosomes in daughter cells—that is, 2^2 or 2 x 2 = 4 possibilities. And in humans there are 2^{23} different possible combinations, two of each chromosome and twenty-three different chromosomes—or 2 x 2 x 2 x 2 x 2 x 2 x 2 x 2 x 2 x 2 x 2 x 2 x 2 x 2 x 2 x 2 x 2 x 2 x 2 x 2 x 2 x 2 x 2 = almost 8.4 million possible combinations for all twenty-three chromosomes.

This random distribution of paired chromosomes is called independent assortment of chromosomes. Independent assortment occurs separately for each of the twenty-three different chromosomes.

Since both parents must contribute genetic material to a child, children will always share traits with their mothers and fathers. Independent assortment explains how we can share traits with all four of our grandparents. If chromosomes were kept as sets, a child would either inherit the grand-paternal or grand-maternal set, not a mixture. Independent assortment provides genetic variability because of the mixing of the chromosome sets in different combinations not only from generation to generation but also from sibling to sibling.

Recombination

The genes on each chromosome are also mixed during the production of eggs and sperm. The mixing of individual genes provides for even greater variation in the genetic traits inherited as a set, helping to make all individuals genetically different except for identical twins. The process of trading genes is called recombination.

Recombination is a precise exchange of genetic material that occurs before the first cell division of meiosis. Recombination occurs when the chromosomes of a pair come into close contact with each other. The two chromosomes of a pair are often called "homologs." For example, the two

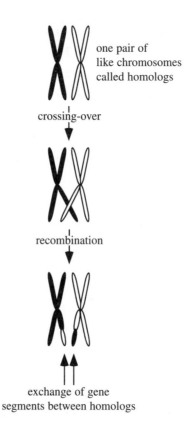

FIGURE 9.2 Diagram showing how recombination occurs during meiosis. Recombination occurs between the members of a pair of chromosomes known as homologs. Genes from the end of one chromosome are swapped with the genes from the homolog, the other chromosome of the pair. Under normal circumstances recombination occurs between like chromosomes, such as chromosome 1 swapping with chromosome 1. Recombination that occurs between dissimilar chromosomes, such as chromosome 13 swapping with chromosome 14, is called a "translocation." Translocations can result in a genetic imbalance if genetic material is gained or lost.

chromosome 1s of a cell are homologs. When recombination happens, the homologs trade information with each other in a kind of swap meet. The DNA strands break and join with other strands of the same chromosome pair. Recombination is also sometimes called "crossing-over."

Normally, the genes remain in the same order and on the same number chromosome, but the genes carried on each of the parent's chromosomes may be swapped with the genes on the other chromosome of that parent. Genes are still passed from one generation to the next through the inheritance of chromosomes, but the genes may occur in some new chromosomal context due to recombination.

The new genetic context can be important when many genes are required to work together to perform a particular task. For example, if a genetic trait is influenced by many genes, shuffling of the genes makes for constantly changing sets of genes from one generation to the next. This means that the genes that worked together to make a trait in one person may not be inherited as a group in that person's children, and the children may show a different likelihood of developing the same trait.

Independent assortment and recombination can be confusing, but they are important to mention because they describe two ways that variation can occur within the species. Also, errors in either independent assortment or recombination can be the cause of alterations in the content of the genetic information. Remember, the inaccurate assortment of chromosomes can cause aneuploid cells because of improper numbers of chromosomes being distributed to sperm and eggs. Errors in recombination caused by misalignment of chromosomes or unbalanced exchanges during crossing-over can result in lost or rearranged genetic material such as deletions, duplications, or other rearrangements of chromosomes. These processes are clinically significant because, as will be described in more detail in Chapter 10, there are genetic diseases that are caused by errors in both independent assortment and recombination.

While the focus of this chapter has been genetic variability among individuals, it is important to point out that, as human beings, we are also genetically very similar. The genetic variables that make us unique are minuscule when compared to our similarities as a species.

CHAPTER TEN

Patterns of Inheritance

One of the many questions that individuals, especially parents, ask when they have been diagnosed with a genetic disease is about the risk that the disorder could happen again in their children or other family members. To answer this question, it is important to understand how a mutation in a gene causes disease. As we have already learned, hereditary genetic diseases can appear when a mutation in a gene is passed from a parent to a child. But having a mutation in a gene does not always mean genetic disease. This chapter and the next will describe the ways in which genetic mutations are manifest as genetic disease.

The pattern of inheritance of a genetic disease is a descriptive term that identifies the way carriers of a gene mutation are affected and the way that they pass the disease risk to their children. There are several different categories for patterns of inheritance. The pattern of inheritance for a genetic disease is determined experimentally by studying family histories of patients with the disease.

Knowing the pattern of inheritance of a genetic disease is very important for genetic counseling. In order to fully assess a family affected by a genetic disease, geneticists and genetic counselors will frequently ask patients for information about their family's medical history. Geneticists sometimes need to know who else in the family is affected and by what types of symptoms in order to precisely diagnose the patient. Learning about a family's medical history can also help determine how a disease is being transmitted through a family and who else in the family is at risk for inheriting or developing the disease.

The tool that geneticists use to diagram a family is called a "pedigree." A pedigree is a drawing of a family tree. As we proceed through the examples in this chapter, sample pedigrees of fictitious families will be used to help illustrate the different patterns of inheritance.

For many genetic diseases, the patterns of inheritance are well defined and genetic counseling is fairly straightforward. In other diseases, however, inheritance may be complex or not yet well understood. Under these circumstances, diagnosis and prediction of risk can become complicated.

Each of the classifications that follow assumes that the genetic defect does not prevent reproduction. Individuals who cannot have children obviously cannot pass on mutations. If future technologies make reproduction possible in individuals where it was not previously achievable, then medical questions will inevitably arise regarding the risk of passing certain mutations and diseases to children.

In contrast to inherited genetic disease, some genetic diseases result when a new mutation develops in a person—a mutation that was not present in that person's parents. This type of disease, while genetic, is not inherited. Nonhereditary genetic disease will be discussed in more detail in the next chapter.

Autosomal vs. Sex-Linked Inheritance

"Autosomal inheritance" describes diseases that occur due to mutations in genes carried on an autosome chromosome—that is, any one of chromosomes 1 through 22. Remember, the 23rd chromosome pair, the X and Y chromosomes, is the one that determines sex. Autosome chromosomes do not include the sex chromosomes. Sex-linked inheritance is a separate form of inheritance.

Since both males and females carry chromosomes 1 through 22, both males and females can be affected by autosomal diseases. In addition, both males and females can pass on a mutation in an autosomal gene to children by passing the chromosome carrying the mutated gene to a child. Remember, there are two of each autosomal chromosome per cell. The choice of which one of a pair of chromosomes is delivered to a sperm or egg is random. As a result, each autosomal chromosome and each autosomal mutation has a 50 percent chance of being passed to a child.

"X-linked inheritance," sometimes called "sex-linked inheritance," describes diseases that occur due to mutations in genes carried on the X chromosome. Since both males and females carry at least one X chromosome, both males and females can be affected by X-linked diseases. For women, who carry two X chromosomes, each X chromosome of the pair in a female has a 50 percent chance of being passed to each child. As a result, a woman that carries a normal gene on one X chromosome and a mutated gene on her other X chromosome has a 50 percent chance of passing the mutated gene to each child.

The single X chromosome of a male will be passed to all of his daughters because if the father gives an X chromosome, the child is a daughter. If the X chromosome of a male carries a gene with a mutation, all of his daughters will inherit the mutated gene. The X chromosome of a male will not be passed to any of his sons because sons inherit the father's Y chromosome. Therefore, only daughters are at risk of inheriting an X chromosome gene mutation from their father.

"Y-linked inheritance" describes genetic traits that occur due to mutations in genes carried on the Y chromosome. Since women carry two X chromosomes and do not carry a Y chromosome, Y-linked traits or disease will only be found in men and can only be passed from fathers to sons.

A few genes have recently been discovered on the Y chromosome. Of the genes found so far, many are believed to be important in male sexual development. Other genes on the Y chromosome are thought to be involved in the regulation of gene expression or in specific male traits such as tooth size.

Since many Y-linked genes are believed to be involved in male sexual development and sperm production, gene mutations on the Y chromosome may sometimes interfere with fertility. Infertile males will obviously not pass a Y-linked mutated gene to a son without some form of medical intervention. As more genes on the Y chromosome are characterized and understood, a number of other male traits may soon be defined as Y-linked.

Mitochondrial Inheritance or Maternal Inheritance

Besides the nucleus of the cell, where the chromosomal DNA resides, there is one other location in the cell where DNA can be found. It is within a membrane-bound structure contained inside cells called a "mitochondrion."

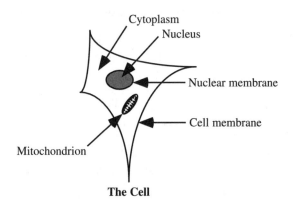

The Cell

FIGURE 10.1 A cell surrounded by a cell membrane. Inside the cytoplasm of the cell is a membrane-bound compartment called the nucleus and a membrane-bound compartment called a mitochondrion. There are usually many mitochondria in a single cell.

Mitochondria are found within the cytoplasm of cells and a single cell may contain many mitochondria. In humans, mitochondria contain a circular DNA molecule of slightly more than 16,000 base pairs. A single mitochondrion can contain several DNA molecules. The mitochondrial DNA encodes about a dozen proteins and a number of RNAs. The function of the mitochondrion is to produce energy for the cell to use in carrying out its tasks. Of the many mitochondria that can be carried in a single cell, some may carry DNA mutations. Mitochondria that carry DNA mutations are one cause of mitochondrial genetic diseases.

Mitochondria are passed from parents to children only through eggs, not through sperm. As a result, defects in mitochondrial genes are passed from mothers to their children. Since sperm do not contribute mitochondria to a child, mitochondrial genes are not generally believed to be passed from fathers to any of their children. This is why mitochondrial inheritance of genetic diseases is sometimes also called "maternal inheritance." In a family tree with a mitochondrially inherited disease, women affected by a mitochondrial disease will have affected children, both male and female. Men affected by the same disease will generally not have affected children.

The severity of genetic disease due to mitochondrial mutations can be highly variable and is dependent upon both the number of mutated mitochondria present in a cell and the mitochondrial gene that carries a mutation. Having many mutated mitochondria in a cell and fewer normal mitochondria could signal more severe disease. The more vital the mutated gene is to proper mitochondrial function, the more devastating the impact of the mutation will be and the more severe the disease may be. In addition, the ratio of normal to mutated mitochondria can vary significantly among different eggs and between the different organs and tissues of any individual. This variability can cause differences in disease severity within the members of a family. Mitochondrial encephalopathy, lactic acidosis, and stroke-like episodes, or MELAS, and Leber's hereditary optic neuropathy are examples of mitochondrial genetic diseases.

At present, scientists do not clearly understand the manner by which mitochondria are produced and distributed to daughter cells during meiosis or mitosis. It is thought that a woman whose eggs carry some mutant and some normal mitochondria may pass a variable ratio of mutant to normal mitochondria to each child. Children who inherit mostly normal mitochondrial DNA may be more mildly affected than children who inherit fewer normal mitochondria. Children who inherit mostly mutated mitochondrial DNA may be very severely affected. It is not yet possible to predict accurately the mitochondrial makeup of any given egg. It is also not yet possible to predict how mitochondria will be distributed to different organs and tissues during the growth and development of any individual.

Such ambiguities in the transmission of mitochondria from mothers to children and from cell to cell make predictions of recurrence risk and severity in mitochondrial diseases very complex. Good estimates of risk of the disease in children are difficult to provide because we are unable to predict how normal and mutated mitochondria are distributed to eggs during meiosis. It

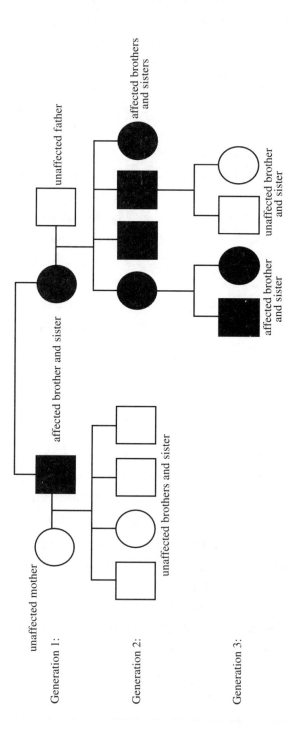

FIGURE 10.2 Pedigree of a fictitious family affected by a mitochondrial or maternally inherited genetic disease. Women are drawn as circles. Men are drawn as squares. Open circles represent unaffected women while shaded circles represent women affected by the disease. Open squares represent unaffected men while shaded squares represent men affected by the disease. Couples are drawn directly connected by a single straight line. Brothers and sisters are connected by a horizontal line above their symbols with vertical lines dropping down to their symbols. For simplicity, the partners of the individuals in generation 2 who are parents have not been drawn, but they should be considered to be unaffected. Note that affected men do not pass the disease to their children but affected women do.

may also be difficult to predict how severely a child might be affected because we cannot always predict how mutated mitochondria will be distributed to the various tissues of the body. New research studies are currently being conducted that are teaching us about how mitochondria are divided and assorted during meiosis and mitosis. The results of these studies may someday provide doctors and genetic counselors with more reliable ways to predict the risk and severity of mitochondrial disease in children of affected individuals.

Dominant vs. Recessive Inheritance

Before considering other aspects of genetic inheritance, it is important to remember that normal human cells carry two copies of each autosomal chromosome (chromosomes 1 through 22) and either two X chromosomes (in females) or an X and a Y chromosome (in males). As such, normal cells carry two copies of all autosomal genes. Females carry two copies of X-linked genes because they carry two X chromosomes. Males carry one copy of X-linked and one copy of Y-linked genes because they carry one of each of those chromosomes.

Just as chromosomes are referred to in pairs, genes are also referred to in pairs. Remember that the different members of a chromosome pair are called homologs. However, the different members of a gene pair are called "alleles." The way in which the alleles of a gene pair interact with one another is important for understanding how genetic diseases appear in families.

"Dominant inheritance" describes a pattern of inheritance in which a genetic disease occurs in an individual who has inherited a mutation in a single gene. In other words, in dominant diseases, if an individual has just one allele of a particular gene with a mutation in it, some form of the genetic disorder is present in the individual.

Dominantly inherited diseases are often present in many generations of a family. The affected individual will frequently have an affected parent, grandparent, great grandparent, and so on. In some cases, however, if the affected individual represents a new mutation, that individual will be the first affected person in the family. This circumstance will be discussed in more detail in the next chapter.

For diseases caused by dominant mutations, if there is a second copy of the gene in the cell—for instance, when the mutated gene is on an autosomal chromosome—that second gene may or may not carry a mutation. In some dominant diseases, where a second mutated gene is also present, the individual may be much more severely affected because of an additive effect of the mutations. For example, in achondroplasia, an autosomal dominant form of dwarfism, if an individual carries two achondroplasia genes, that individual is generally much more severely affected than an individual who has one achondroplasia gene and one normal gene. This is because if both genes are altered, both genes produce a defective protein. Individuals in whom both genes are altered make no normal protein. Alternatively, if one gene carries a mutation and the other does not, then some normal protein will be made. Individuals with two achondroplasia genes usually die shortly after birth, whereas individuals with only one achondroplasia gene and one normal gene can live fairly normal life spans.

Since different genes perform different functions, the specific genetic disease and the characteristics of the disease will depend upon the gene in which there is a mutation. There are already many dominantly inherited genetic diseases for which the genes responsible are known and for which common mutations have been characterized.

The risks for passing dominant diseases to children will depend upon whether or not the mutated gene is carried on the X chromosome or on an autosome, and whether or not the parent carries one or two mutated genes. Some of the more specific aspects of dominant genetic disease transmission will be discussed later in this chapter under "autosomal dominant" and "X-linked dominant."

"Recessive inheritance" describes a pattern of inheritance in which a genetic disease occurs only in individuals who lack a normal copy of a particular gene. In other words, if a cell carries a single normal copy of a particular gene, the individual would be without symptoms of the disease. Individuals carrying only mutated copies of a particular gene, with no normal copies of the gene, would be affected by and exhibit symptoms of the disease. Cystic fibrosis (CF) and Tay-Sachs disease are examples of recessive diseases.

The specific genetic disease present and its characteristics will depend on the gene in which there is a mutation. There are already many recessively inherited genetic diseases for which the genes responsible are known and for which common mutations have been characterized.

Unaffected carriers of recessive genetic diseases are persons who have two copies of a particular gene, one with a mutation and one without. Unaffected carriers of recessive mutations have a 50 percent chance of passing the mutation, but not the disease, to a child. There is also a 50 percent chance that each child will not inherit the mutation. The child will inherit the mutation if the child inherits the chromosome carrying the altered gene, but if the child also inherits a normal copy of that gene from the other parent, the child will not be affected by the disease.

Recessive genetic diseases are commonly seen in families as an affected child born to unaffected parents who had no reason to suspect that they were carriers for a genetic disease. Sometimes though, there may be siblings, cousins, aunts, or uncles affected by the same genetic disease, representing a family history of the disease.

The risks for passing recessive genetic diseases to children will also depend upon whether the disease gene is carried on an autosome or the X chromosome. Some of the more specific aspects of recessive genetic disease transmission will be discussed later in this chapter under "autosomal recessive" and "X-linked recessive."

Patterns of Inheritance

When referring to the pattern of inheritance of a genetic disease, two terms are usually employed. The terms "autosomal" or "X-linked" are combined with either of the terms "dominant" or "recessive." Usually, mitochondrial diseases are not referred to as recessive or dominant because their symptoms depend on the presence of mutated mitochondria in a cell, the ratio of normal to mutated mitochondria, and the type of mutation that has occurred.

Autosomal Dominant

"Autosomal dominant inheritance" describes genetic diseases caused by mutations in genes carried on autosomes (chromosomes 1 through 22) that are manifest in individuals with only a single mutated copy of a gene. In most cases of autosomal dominant disease, the second allele of the gene pair is normal, but this is not necessarily so. Achondroplasia, neurofibromatosis, and Marfan syndrome are examples of autosomal dominant diseases. In addition, inherited or familial forms of cancer such as hereditary nonpolyposis coli (HNPCC), familial adenomatous polyposis coli (FAP or APC), and inherited breast cancer generally show an autosomal dominant pattern of inheritance but with reduced penetrance (see Chapter 11).

Autosomal dominant diseases are generally observed across several generations of a family. The affected individual frequently has an affected parent, grandparent, great grandparent, and so on. When the family history is diagrammed as a pedigree, autosomal dominant disease may be seen as the consistent appearance of symptoms in many generations of the family tree.

Now let us consider a common scenario for a family affected by an autosomal dominant disease. In this imaginary family, one parent is affected by the disease while the other is not. In this case, we want to determine the genetic risk for a child of this couple. This child has a risk of inheriting the disease gene from the affected parent, but not from the unaffected parent.

Normally, there are two copies of each autosomal chromosome in a person. The parent affected by autosomal dominant disease will often carry one normal and one mutated gene. We will assume, for this example, that this is the case. As a result, there is a 50 percent chance that the affected parent will pass the mutated gene to any given child. This results in a 50 percent chance for that parent of having an affected child with each new pregnancy, depending upon whether or not the chromosome carrying the altered gene is passed to the child.

If, however, the affected parent has two mutated genes and no normal gene, each child will have a 100 percent chance of being affected, because there is no unaltered gene to be transmitted from the affected parent.

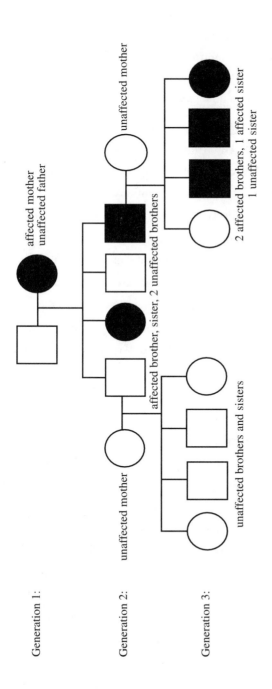

FIGURE 10.3   A diagram representing the pedigree of a fictitious family affected by an autosomal dominant genetic disease. Women are drawn as circles. Men are drawn as squares. Open circles represent unaffected women while shaded circles represent women affected by the disease. Open squares represent unaffected men while shaded squares represent men affected by the disease. Couples are drawn directly connected by a single straight line. Brothers and sisters are connected by a horizontal line above their symbols with vertical lines dropping down to their symbols. Note that both males and females can be affected by an autosomal dominant disease and that the disease can be passed from affected parents to children over several generations.

Now, let us consider a more complicated situation. Assume that both parents are affected by the same autosomal dominant disorder and that both parents carry one normal and one mutated gene. Either parent could pass the mutated gene to a child. As a result, each child of these parents has only a 25 percent chance of being unaffected by the disease. This is because the child could get the disease gene from either parent.

Additionally, each child has a 25 percent chance of being affected with two mutated genes. This is because each child has a 50 percent (one in two) chance of getting a mutated gene from the mother and a 50 percent (one in two) chance of getting a mutated gene from the father, too. Mathematically, one in two times one in two (1/2 x 1/2) equals one in four (1/4) or 25 percent. In some cases such as achondroplasia, individuals who carry two mutated genes are much more severely affected, and that risk is an important consideration for some parents.

Each child of these parents also has a 50 percent chance of being affected but carrying only one mutated gene. That is a 50 percent chance of inheriting the normal gene from one parent and the mutated gene from the other.

Let's simplify this case with an illustration and try to make it easier to understand. To do this, we can break everything down into symbols. With symbols, we can consider the four parental genes as individual units. Each parent has one normal and one mutated gene. As a result, between the two parents there are a total of two normal genes and two mutated genes, one normal and one mutated gene in each parent.

This can be illustrated in a figure known as a Punnett square, as shown in Figure 10-4, where the parental genotypes are written outside the box horizontally and vertically. The possible genotypes of the children are drawn inside the box, using the crosses from outside the box to fill in the columns.

Following along in the figure, if the normal gene is designated "a" and the mutated gene is designated "A" (a dominant disease gene being designated by a capital letter), then we can consider both parents as each carrying an "A" gene and an "a" gene. So the genetic type or "genotype" of each parent can be written "Aa," designating one mutated and one normal gene.

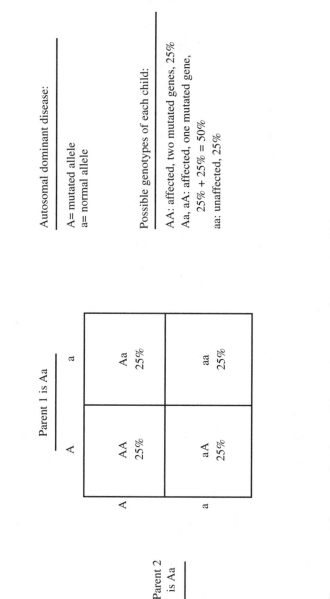

Assume: Parental genotypes are Aa and Aa

Autosomal dominant disease:

A = mutated allele
a = normal allele

Possible genotypes of each child:

AA: affected, two mutated genes, 25%
Aa, aA: affected, one mutated gene,
25% + 25% = 50%
aa: unaffected, 25%

FIGURE 10.4 A Punnett square demonstrating the possible genetic outcomes for each child of a set of parents affected by an autosomal dominant genetic disease. The Punnett square shown here is specific for a case in which each parent carries one gene with a mutation and one normal gene.

Now, assume that parent 1 gives a child the mutated "A" gene. The other parent could give the child either the mutated "A" gene or the normal "a" gene. The possible genotypes of the child are "AA" and "aA." Genotype "AA" would result in an affected child with two mutated genes, and genotype "aA" would result in an affected child with one normal gene and one mutated gene. Each possible genotype could occur with equal likelihood.

Now, assume that parent 1 gives a child the other gene, the normal "a" gene. The other parent can give either the mutated "A" gene or the normal "a" gene. The possible genotypes are "Aa" and "aa." Genotype "Aa" would result in an affected child with one mutated gene and one normal gene, and genotype "aa" would result in an unaffected child. Again, each possible genotype could occur with equal likelihood.

So, in all, there are four possible outcomes for the child: "AA," "aA," "Aa," or "aa." Each would occur with the same likelihood—25 percent. So there is a 25 percent that the child will be affected with two mutated genes or "AA," a 50 percent chance that the child will be affected with one mutated gene (25 percent "aA" plus 25 percent "Aa"), and a 25 percent chance that the child will be unaffected with two normal genes, or "aa."

Autosomal Recessive

"Autosomal recessive inheritance" refers to diseases inherited due to a mutation in genes carried on autosomes (chromosomes 1 through 22) and present only in individuals with mutations in both copies of a particular gene. Individuals who carry only a single copy of a mutation in a truly autosomal recessive gene are unaffected and do not show symptoms of the disease. CF and Tay-Sachs disease are examples of autosomal recessive diseases.

Autosomal recessive diseases frequently appear in families as an affected child born to unaffected parents. This occurs when both parents are carriers of a mutated gene. Unaffected carriers of autosomal recessive diseases, such as the individuals in generation 1 of Figure 10.5, carry one gene with a mutation and one normal gene. Since unaffected carriers of autosomal recessive genetic diseases generally do not show symptoms of the disease

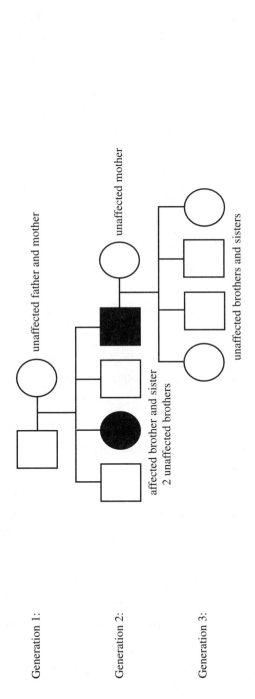

FIGURE 10.5   A diagram representing the pedigree of a fictitious family affected by an autosomal recessive genetic disease. Women are drawn as circles. Men are drawn as squares. Open circles represent unaffected women while shaded circles represent women affected by the disease. Open squares represent unaffected men while shaded squares represent men affected by the disease. Couples are drawn directly connected by a single straight line. Brothers and sisters are connected by a horizontal line above their symbols with vertical lines dropping down to their symbols. Note that both males and females can be affected by an autosomal recessive disease and that the disease appears as affected children born to unaffected parents.

in question, they may have no reason to suspect that they are carriers of a genetic disease, unless there is a family history.

Unaffected carriers of autosomal recessive mutations have a one in two, or 50 percent, chance of passing the mutated gene, but not the disease, to a child. Unaffected carrier couples, where both partners are unaffected carriers of the same recessive disease, have a one in four, or 25 percent, chance of having an affected child with each pregnancy (one in two chance that the child gets a mutated gene from one parent times a one in two chance that the child also gets a mutated gene from the other parent: $1/2 \times 1/2 = 1/4$, or 25 percent).

This circumstance can also be visualized using a Punnett square. In the case of recessive diseases, however, geneticists use a lower case letter to designate the affected gene. As such, the "a" is associated with the recessive disease, while the unaffected dominant genes are designated by capital letters. This is diagrammed in Figure 10-6, where the parental genotypes are written outside the box horizontally and vertically. The possible genotypes of the children are drawn inside the box, using the crosses from outside the box to fill in the columns.

So in this case, the "A" is the normal gene and both parents are "Aa," unaffected carriers. There are four possible outcomes for each child as follows. If parent 1 gives the child a normal "A" gene, then the second parent can give either the normal "A" gene or the mutated "a" gene. The possible genotypes of the child are "AA" and "aA." Each outcome will carry the same likelihood of occurrence.

If parent 1 gives the child a mutated "a" gene, then the second parent can give either the normal "A" gene or the mutated "a" gene. The possible genotypes of the child here are "Aa" and "aa." Each outcome will carry the same likelihood of occurrence.

As a result, the four possible outcomes for each child will be "AA," "aA," "Aa," or "aa." Each child will have a 25 percent chance of being "AA," an unaffected non-carrier; a 50 percent chance of being "Aa," an unaffected carrier (25 percent chance of being "Aa" plus 25 percent chance of being "aA"); and a 25 percent chance of being "aa," affected.

Assume: Parental genotypes are Aa and Aa

Autosomal recessive disease:

A= normal allele
a= mutated allele

Possible genotypes of each child:

AA: unaffected, noncarrier, 25%
Aa, aA: unaffected, carrier, 25% + 25% = 50%
aa: affected, 25%

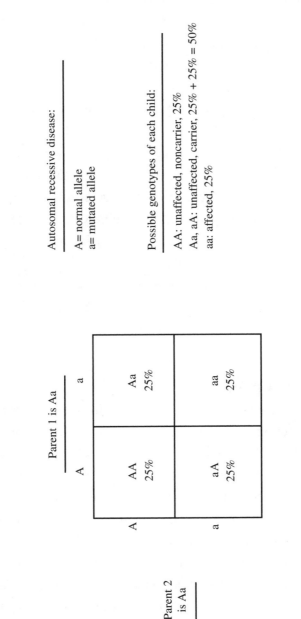

Parent 1 is Aa

	A	a
A	AA 25%	Aa 25%
a	aA 25%	aa 25%

Parent 2
is Aa

FIGURE 10.6 A Punnett square demonstrating the possible genetic outcomes for each child of a set of parents who are both unaffected carriers for the same autosomal recessive disease. Unaffected carriers of autosomal recessive genetic diseases have one gene with a mutation and one normal gene.

Individuals who are affected by autosomal recessive diseases will always pass a mutation to their children because they have no normal gene to contribute. However, a child will only be affected by the disease if the other parent is either affected or an unaffected carrier and the child inherits a mutation from that parent as well.

If one parent is affected by an autosomal recessive disease and the second parent is an unaffected carrier, then each child has a 50 percent chance of being affected. This is so because the child will always inherit a mutated gene from the affected parent since that parent has no unaffected gene to give. But the other parent has two genes to give, one normal and one with a mutation. As such, the child will only be affected if he or she inherits the mutated gene from the unaffected carrier parent. This will occur with a 50 percent likelihood.

If, however, both parents are affected by the same autosomal recessive disease, all the children of the couple will be affected because neither parent has an unaffected gene to contribute to a child.

X-Linked Dominant

"X-linked dominant inheritance" describes diseases inherited due to mutations in genes on the X chromosome that are manifest in carrier individuals regardless of the number of X chromosomes the person has. Therefore, diseases that show X-linked dominant inheritance can be observed in both male and female carriers of the mutation. In X-linked dominant diseases, the copy of the gene on the second X chromosome of females may or may not carry a mutation.

X-linked dominant genetic disease can be observed across several generations of a family. The affected individual may have an affected parent, grandparent, great grandparent, and so on. However, for some X-linked dominant disorders, affected males are not observed—only affected females are seen. These diseases, such as incontinentia pigmenti, are thought to be lethal to males in early development, explaining why no affected males and only affected females with one normal and one mutated gene are seen. It is

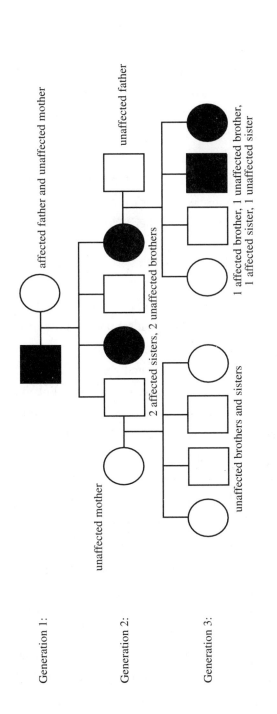

Generation 1:

affected father and unaffected mother

unaffected mother

Generation 2:

unaffected father

2 affected sisters, 2 unaffected brothers

Generation 3:

unaffected brothers and sisters

1 affected brother, 1 unaffected brother,
1 affected sister, 1 unaffected sister

FIGURE 10.7 A diagram representing the pedigree of a fictitious family affected by an X-linked dominant genetic disease. Women are drawn as circles. Men are drawn as squares. Open circles represent unaffected women while shaded circles represent women affected by the disease. Open squares represent unaffected men while shaded squares represent men affected by the disease. Couples are drawn directly connected by a single straight line. Brothers and sisters are connected by a horizontal line above their symbols with vertical lines dropping down to their symbols. Note that both males and females can be affected by an X-linked dominant disease and that the disease is passed from fathers only to daughters and from mothers to both sons and daughters.

thought that the presence of one normal gene is necessary and sufficient to rescue the embryo.

Women affected by X-linked dominant diseases who carry one normal and one mutated gene have a 50 percent chance of passing the disease to each child—daughter or son—depending upon whether the X chromosome carrying the mutation is passed. Affected females who carry two mutated alleles will always pass a mutated gene to their children because they do not have a normal gene to contribute.

Males affected by X-linked dominant diseases will always pass the disease to their daughters because daughters must inherit the father's X chromosome. X-linked dominant diseases will never be passed from affected fathers to sons because sons inherit the father's Y chromosome, not the X.

X-Linked Recessive

"X-linked recessive inheritance" describes diseases inherited due to mutations in genes on the X chromosome that are present primarily in males because males carry only one X chromosome. Female carriers of X-linked recessive diseases will often have one mutated gene and one normal gene and will, in the majority of cases, not show symptoms of X-linked recessive diseases. If, however, a female carries X-linked recessive mutations in both copies of the same gene, then she would be predicted to be affected by the disease. Duchenne muscular dystrophy and Lesch-Nyhan syndrome are examples of X-linked recessive diseases.

X-linked recessive genetic diseases are generally observed in families as affected males born to unaffected mothers. Sometimes, X-linked recessive genetic diseases can be seen in several generations of a family as affected uncles and nephews, affected boys with affected grandfathers or great grandfathers, or in several branches of the family tree as affected male cousins. However, in many cases, the affected male is the first affected individual to be diagnosed in a family.

X-linked color blindness is a non-disease example of a common human trait that is inherited in an X-linked recessive manner. As a result, color blindness

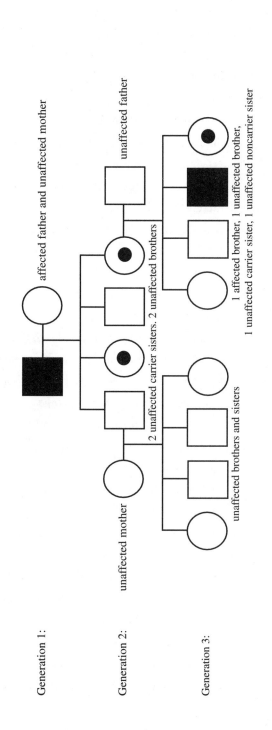

Generation 1:

affected father and unaffected mother

Generation 2:

unaffected father

unaffected mother

2 unaffected carrier sisters, 2 unaffected brothers

Generation 3:

unaffected brothers and sisters

1 affected brother, 1 unaffected brother,
1 unaffected carrier sister, 1 unaffected noncarrier sister

FIGURE 10.8 A diagram representing the pedigree of a fictitious family affected by an X-linked recessive genetic disease. Women are drawn as circles. Men are drawn as squares. Open circles represent unaffected noncarrier women while circles with dots in the center represent women who are unaffected carriers of the disease. Open squares represent unaffected men while shaded squares represent men affected by the disease. Couples are drawn directly connected by a single straight line. Brothers and sisters are connected by a horizontal line above their symbols with vertical lines dropping down to their symbols. Note that only males are affected by X-linked recessive diseases, and that the disease is passed from affected fathers to unaffected carrier daughters and from unaffected carrier mothers to affected sons and unaffected carrier daughters. Notice also how the disease appears to skip a generation, appearing in a grandfather and grandsons but not in the intervening generation.

is most often seen in males. But color blindness is fairly common, and females can sometimes be color blind. Females can be color blind if they carry a color blindness gene on both of their X chromosomes. X-linked color blindness is seen in about 8 percent of males and less than 1 percent of females.

X-linked recessive diseases that are carried by unaffected females with one normal and one mutated gene have a 50 percent chance of being passed to each child. If the child is a son, there is a 50 percent chance that he will be affected by the disease, depending upon whether he inherits the X chromosome carrying the altered gene. If the child is a daughter, she has a 50 percent chance of being a carrier, depending on which of the two X chromosomes she inherits.

If a woman is affected by an X-linked recessive disease because she carries two mutated genes, she will pass the mutation to all of her children because she has no unaffected gene to contribute. As a result, all of her sons will be affected, and all of her daughters will be carriers.

Males affected with X-linked recessive diseases will pass the mutated gene to all of their daughters, because the father has just the one X chromosome to pass to a daughter. The daughters would generally only be affected if they also inherit a mutation from their mothers. Males affected with X-linked recessive diseases would never pass the mutation to any of their sons, because sons inherit their father's Y chromosome, not their father's X chromosome.

In a slightly more complicated case, if an X-linked recessive trait or disease is very common, a son could inherit a mutation from his carrier mother, while also having an affected father. Since the mother would be unaffected, it might appear that the son got the disease from his father, even though this would not actually be the case.

Sometimes, females can show symptoms of X-linked recessive diseases. One way this can happen is if a female has mutations in both copies of the gene. Another way is if a female is missing all or a portion of an X chromosome. For example, in Turner syndrome, a female will often carry only one X chromosome. The other X chromosome will not be present. If her one X chromosome also carries a mutation in a gene, the affected female can have both Turner syndrome and the genetic disease for which she carries a mutation. Rarely, females can have some other complicated rearrangement of X chromosome material such as a translocation. A translocation, which was explained more fully in Chapter 9, is an exchange of genetic material between unlike or nonhomologous chromosomes. If a translocation occurs in a female with a net loss of X chromosome material, expression of an X-linked recessive disease may occur.

In rare cases, there is another way that females can show symptoms of X-linked recessive diseases without carrying mutations in both copies of the gene and without having Turner syndrome. This can be explained by a process called "nonrandom X inactivation." Remember that females carry two X chromosomes and males carry only one. But even though females have twice as many X chromosomes as males, they do not express a double dose of all the X chromosome genes.

For most X-linked genes, females show the same level of expression of those genes as do males who only carry one X chromosome. Initially, this was very confusing, but scientists have learned that only one of the X chromosomes in female cells expresses all of its genes. The other X chromosome is inactivated, or switched off, early in development. Most of the genes from the inactivated X chromosome are not expressed (transcribed), although there are some exceptions.

The X chromosome that is switched off is randomly chosen early in development. As a result, some cells of females express genes from the X chromosome that came from the mother and other cells express genes from the X chromosome that came from the father. Since the inactivation of an X chromosome is random, theoretically, half of a female's cells should express genes from one X chromosome, while the other half of her cells express genes from the other X chromosome.

The choice of the inactive X is maintained for all future descendants of a given cell, throughout countless mitoses. That is, once a cell chooses to inactivate a particular X chromosome, all of its future daughter cells, except egg cells, also inactivate that same X chromosome.

The result of truly randomized X inactivation would be that females carrying an X-linked recessive mutation should have a sufficient number of cells expressing the normal gene, about half, to compensate for the cells expressing the mutated gene. But X inactivation is not always entirely random. Especially in the individual tissues of a female, predominant inactivation of a particular X chromosome is sometimes seen.

If significantly more than half of the cells of a female, or any of her tissues, express genes from only one X chromosome, then X inactivation is said to be nonrandom. If the predominantly active X chromosome carries a gene with a mutation, then there may be physical effects from the mutation. These effects would be seen as symptoms of an X-linked recessive disease in a female. Symptoms occur because of the large number of cells that express the mutated gene. Many female cases of X-linked recessive genetic diseases are now thought to be caused by nonrandom X inactivation. Future research is expected to provide more detailed information about the genetic and biological mechanisms behind skewing of X inactivation in females.

Chromosomal Disorders

Alterations in chromosomes that do not interfere with the reproductive capabilities of the carrier can sometimes be passed to future generations. Chromosomal alterations are inherited by offspring who inherit the altered chromosome, and since there are two of each chromosome, any given chromosome of a pair has a 50 percent chance of being passed to each child.

However, very often chromosomal alterations are fairly devastating if not lethal for the affected individual and instead of being passed from parent to child, they appear as new mutations that occurred during meiosis of the sperm or egg, or during the growth and development of the affected child. By definition, these new mutations are not found in the parents of the affected child. As such, truly new mutations generally carry a very low recurrence risk because the parents do not carry the mutation. New mutation genetic disease is discussed in more detail in the next chapter. If however, the alteration exists in some percentage of the parent's germ cells (the sperm or egg precursors), then there may be a risk for a parent of having another affected child. This circumstance is called "gonadal mosaicism" and will also be discussed in more detail in the next chapter.

There are several genetic diseases that have been determined to be caused by specific, characteristic chromosomal alterations. The symptoms and severity of these diseases depend upon the precise chromosomal alteration and the genes disrupted.

Just like gene mutations, chromosomal alterations can take several forms. Chromosomes can have deletions, where part of a chromosome is missing. Deletions can sometimes occur in the middle of a chromosome. These deletions are called "interstitial deletions" and the ends of the chromosome are generally intact with some amount of material from the midsection of the chromosome missing. Deletions can also sometimes occur at the ends of the chromosome. These deletions are called "terminal deletions" and the missing material is from one end of the chromosome. Prader-Willi and Angelman syndromes are examples of genetic diseases frequently caused by deletions in a particular interstitial region of chromosome 15.

Chromosomes can have duplications where part of a chromosome occurs more times than it normally would. Duplications of chromosomes also generally involve duplication of all or parts of some number of genes.

Chromosomes can have insertion mutations where material occurs in a chromosome that is not normally there. Such foreign genetic material can come from another chromosome or from some external source.

Chromosomes can carry inversions where a segment of the chromosome is flipped end for end. The size, section, and chromosome involved in an inversion will generally have an important impact on the effect of the alteration.

Chromosomes can also carry translocations wherein a piece of one chromosome is transferred to another chromosome and attached to it. If segments from two chromosomes are swapped for each other, it is called a "reciprocal translocation." If a translocation occurs with no net loss of genetic material, the translocation is said to be a "balanced translocation."

Sometimes, carriers of balanced translocations and inversions are completely normal and do not even know they carry a chromosomal alteration until they try to have children. In such cases, it is only upon testing due to reproductive difficulties, multiple miscarriages, or infertility that the translocation is discovered.

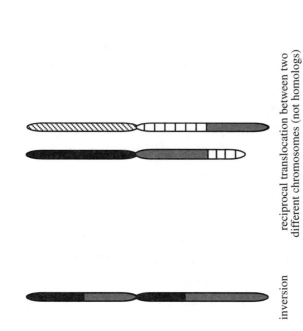

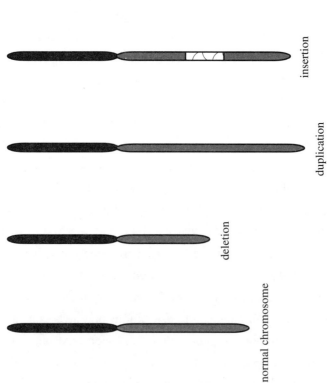

FIGURE 10.9 Diagram showing a schematic representation of the different types of chromosomal alterations.

A common example of a genetic disease caused by a translocation is Down syndrome. As discussed in a previous chapter, most cases of Down syndrome are caused by the presence of an extra whole chromosome 21—where individuals carry forty-seven instead of forty-six chromosomes, with three chromosome 21s. But Down syndrome can also be caused by a translocation where all or part of chromosome 21 is attached to another chromosome. In these cases, the affected individual carries the additional chromosome 21 material stuck onto another chromosome. The translocation of the chromosome 21 material to another chromosome results in three copies of chromosome 21 material occurring within the cell, but since the extra material is stuck onto another chromosome and not free standing, the patient still has forty-six chromosomes.

The distinction between Down syndrome caused by an extra chromosome and Down syndrome caused by a translocation inherited from a carrier parent is important for estimating the risk that a parent might have another affected child. For Down syndrome caused by an extra chromosome there is a much lower risk of having another affected child than there is for Down syndrome caused by a parentally carried balanced translocation. Parents carrying a translocation involving chromosome 21 generally have a much greater risk of having another child affected by Down syndrome. The age of the mother is also an important consideration in estimating recurrence risk for Down syndrome.

Important Considerations
About the Calculation of Genetic Risk

As you have seen here, the calculation of genetic risk is not a simple task. Each family and each genetic disease is specific and unique, and there are many factors that can complicate the calculation of genetic risk. As difficult as the examples given here may seem to be, they are actually very simplified and take into account few if any extenuating circumstances.

In reality, the calculation of genetic risk is frequently complicated by a number of factors. For example, sometimes the genetic status of the parents may be difficult to determine, making a parent's carrier status unclear and a child's risk difficult to determine.

Sometimes the same clinical disease can be caused by mutations in any one of several different genes, making the classification of a pattern of inheritance unreliable without extensive medical evaluation of patients and family histories. And sometimes, even then, classification of a pattern of inheritance is not clear.

Family history and ethnicity can also affect risk predictions dramatically.

Because of the difficulties in characterizing genetic diseases, it is not advisable for individuals to try to calculate genetic risks for themselves. The examples shown in this chapter are for illustrative purposes only and are provided to give individuals an idea of how genetic risks are calculated. It would be impossible to list here all of the possible exceptions that could occur, exceptions that could result in errors in the calculations if not properly considered.

It is very important that patients, families, and individuals who have a family history or prior occurrence of a genetic disease or concerns for inheritance or transmission of a genetic disease see a qualified genetics professional. Qualified medical consultation is vital to assuring that the diagnosis of the disease and the calculation of genetic risks for relatives and offspring are accurate.

When consulting about genetic disease, patients should ask their doctors for a clear diagnosis, a description of the pattern of inheritance of the disease, and any exceptions or special conditions that might be relevant. It is important that patients try to understand fully the implications and circumstances of their medical conditions. Understanding the basics will help patients make informed choices about their own medical options and participate in their own treatment and the management of their family's medical needs.

Sometimes genetic diseases interfere with the reproductive capabilities of the affected individual. As such, the calculation of genetic risks for individuals who are not able to reproduce is not relevant.

Sometimes the severity of a genetic disease can vary among members of a family. In these cases, the medical evaluation of additional family members may be of interest to patients and families, particularly if there is a chance that unaffected carriers may exist within the family or if there is a chance that there are mildly affected individuals who may have the disease and not realize it. Such individuals, though not clinically affected, can still be at risk for transmitting the disease to their children.

Finally, it is important to remember that each pregnancy is a new situation for inheritance of chromosomes and genes. Risk calculations for pregnancy outcome are made for each pregnancy individually. For example, just because a couple with a one in four risk of having a child affected by an autosomal recessive disease has one affected child already, it does not mean that the next three children will be normal. Alternatively, if a couple with a one in four risk of having a child affected by an autosomal recessive disease has three unaffected children, it does not mean that the next child will necessarily be affected. There is no compensation for outcomes in genetics. The one in four risk applies to each new pregnancy. The same holds true for the risk of inheriting dominant diseases: Each new pregnancy is a new risk calculation, independent of any and all previous outcomes.

As is common in biology, there are exceptions to many rules, and some diseases do not fit neatly into a specific category. For example, for a disease to be truly recessive, carriers would never show symptoms. For a disease to be truly dominant, individuals carrying one or two copies of a mutated gene should be equally severely affected. Instead, some diseases fall into an intermediate category and can be more difficult to describe. Many of the exceptions to the above rules are discussed in the next chapter. Individuals should be aware of the possibility of these exceptions and seek qualified medical consultation before drawing any of their own conclusions.

CHAPTER ELEVEN

Complex Patterns
of Inheritance

In addition to those introduced in the previous chapter, there are a number of terms patients may hear in genetic counseling situations. Many of these terms, their meanings, and their implications for patients and families will be discussed in this chapter.

Sporadic or New Mutation Genetic Disease

Some genetic diseases show up in what are called "sporadic" cases. Sporadic diseases can be caused by either chromosomal or single gene defects. In sporadic or "new mutation" genetic disease, the affected individual is the first affected individual observed in a family. Sporadic or new mutation genetic diseases are a good example of how genetic disease and inherited disease can be separated into two distinct entities.

Generally, sporadic or new mutation genetic diseases are the result of mutations that occur during or after transmission of a normal gene from an unaffected parent. Sporadic or new mutation genetic diseases occur as a result of errors in meiosis or mitosis, or DNA damage. In these cases, the disease is genetic because it is caused by an alteration in a gene or genes, but it is not inherited because the defect was not present in the parent. However, once a sporadic genetic disease occurs, the affected individual may be at risk for passing the mutation, and possibly the disease, to his or her children.

Achondroplasia, neurofibromatosis, and Marfan syndrome are examples of autosomal dominant diseases that have a high new mutation rate. Many of the individuals affected by these diseases are born to unaffected parents.

However, it is important to remember that for diseases such as Marfan syndrome in which there is great variability in the severity of the disease, it can often be challenging to determine if the disease is truly a new mutation or if, instead, the patient is just a more severely affected child of a very mildly affected and previously undiagnosed parent.

Generally, new mutation diseases appear as dominant conditions because it is highly unlikely that a new mutation would occur in both copies of a gene, as would be required for a recessive disease. Theoretically, new mutations might occur in a gene where a recessive mutation is inherited from the other parent, although this is probably rare.

For X-linked recessive diseases, a new mutation could occur during transmission of an X chromosome gene from a father to his daughter. The father, who does not carry the mutation, is unaffected. The daughter, who is the new mutation case, might not show symptoms of the disease because of random X inactivation. Yet, the daughter is a carrier and is at risk for passing the disease to a future son and for passing the mutation to a future daughter. These cases of new mutations are more complex than simple single-generation appearance of a new mutation. Such possibilities can make genetic counseling more complex.

Duchenne muscular dystrophy and Hemophilia types A and B are examples of X-linked recessive diseases with relatively high new mutation rates that can show a sporadic or new mutation pattern. In many cases, an affected son is born to a carrier mother where the mother is actually the new mutation case. In these cases, until the birth of the affected son, there may have been no reason to suspect that the mother might be a carrier of a genetic disease. However, if the mother is in fact a carrier, then she is at risk for having additional sons affected by the disease and her daughters are at risk for being carriers of the disease. For this reason, carrier testing of women who have sons affected by X-linked recessive diseases is often needed to accurately assess the risk for future affected children in the family.

Except for X-linked recessive cases as described above, the risk of an unaffected non-carrier parent having a second affected child in sporadic cases is often low because the likelihood of a second new mutation is low. There are exceptions, however, such as gonadal mosaicism.

Gonadal Mosaicism

To help explain gonadal mosaicism, also called germ-line mosaicism, it is helpful to think about the development of an individual. Imagine that a new mutation arises during the growth and development of an individual—after fertilization, but during mitosis and growth. If this occurs after only a few mitotic cell divisions, many cells of the body may carry the mutation. If the mutation occurs later in development, only a few cells may carry the mutation.

When this individual becomes a parent, if some of the cells of the body that carry mutations are germ cells, then sperm or egg cells carrying the mutation could be produced. If some but not all of the germ cells carry the mutation, then more than one sperm or egg could be made that carries the mutation. As a result, more than one affected child can be born to an unaffected parent and recurrence of a disease that appears to be a new mutation can occur. The larger the proportion of germ cells that carry the mutation, the greater the risk of recurrence of the disease in subsequent children.

Diseases that show gonadal mosaicism generally show sporadic appearance but with a slightly higher recurrence risk for additional affected children within a family than would be seen for diseases that do not show gonadal mosaicism. The recurrence risks in diseases that show gonadal mosaicism are calculated experimentally by examining large numbers of families with the disease. The recurrence risks based on gonadal mosaicism can vary with different diseases. Risks for some families may also be slightly higher than the risk for others, depending on the observed rate of recurrence in the family and the estimated proportion of germ cells that carry the new mutation.

Genetic counselors and clinical geneticists can often give reasonable estimates of recurrence risk for diseases that show gonadal mosaicism, but patients should be aware that these are just estimates. Each new pregnancy may carry a similar statistical level of risk and, without further testing of a fetus, estimates are not and cannot be considered assurances of pregnancy outcome. For example, if there is a 1 percent risk of additional children being affected by the disease, just because a family has one affected child does not mean that the next ninety-nine children would be unaffected. The 1 percent risk resets for each new pregnancy.

Gonadal mosaicism has been reported for several diseases, including osteogenesis imperfecta. However, gonadal mosaicism is not seen in all new mutation diseases. The possibility of gonadal mosaicism is often an important consideration for parents when discussing sporadic cases of genetic disease.

Anticipation

"Anticipation" is a term that is used to describe genetic diseases that are passed from parent to child, with more severely affected individuals occurring with each new generation. For example, imagine a family in which great grandmother was very mildly affected and maybe never even diagnosed. Grandpa was diagnosed with the disease but was still pretty mild. Dad was noticeably bothered by the disease, and baby is severely affected.

The genetic basis of anticipation was not understood for many years, and there was some debate about whether it actually existed. Some doctors argued that anticipation might instead be nothing more than normal variation in the severity of a disease, and mildly affected individuals were only noticed when someone else sought medical attention. However, we now know that in many cases anticipation is real.

One genetic cause of anticipation has recently been determined to be unstable DNA sequences within genes that are prone to length variations. These unstable sequences can expand and contract in length during meiosis and mitosis. As the unstable sequences change length, variations in disease severity may be seen.

Frequently, genes and diseases in which anticipation occurs have a three-nucleotide sequence, such as C-A-G or C-G-G, that is repeated several times in a row within the gene. If the sequence expands during meiosis or after fertilization, a parent will carry a certain number of repeats of the three-nucleotide sequence, and the child will carry more repeats. If expansion of the sequence occurs, the child will also have a larger-sized gene. If the expanded length of the three-nucleotide (or trinucleotide) repeat is sufficient to disrupt the function of the protein, genetic disease can result. Infrequently, a reduction or contraction in the length of the repeat is seen from parent to child. In these cases, the child carries fewer consecutive repeats than the parent.

Generally speaking, the longer the repeat, the more devastating the effect on the protein and, consequently, the more severe the disease and the earlier symptoms appear. However, this is only a general trend and not an exact rule. As a result, precise prediction of disease severity and accurate estimation of age of onset based solely on repeat length is not yet possible. Frequently, two patients with similarly sized repeats will have different disease profiles.

In some cases, anticipation can result in a genetic disease that is also inherited as a new mutation. For example, if the repeat length in the parent was short enough not to cause symptoms but expanded to a length of clinical significance in the child, the child may be affected when the parent was not. In these cases, the unaffected parent is said to carry a "premutation."

Alternatively, the disease may just seem to be a new mutation because the parent may be very mildly affected by a short repeat, and it is not until the disease shows up more severely in a child that very mild symptoms are noticed in the parent. This last circumstance is fairly common with diseases that show anticipation, because very mildly affected parents may not notice that they have symptoms of a disease and therefore may not seek medical attention until a severely affected child is born. In these cases, genetic analysis of the parents along with the child may provide additional information for families with regard to disease risk for relatives and future offspring.

Current research is focused on identifying the cellular and genetic factors that influence the likelihood of repeat expansion. The complexities of diseases that show anticipation make medical genetic evaluation and genetic counseling important. Myotonic dystrophy, Huntington disease, and fragile X mental retardation are examples of diseases that show anticipation.

Penetrance and Variability

"Penetrance" refers to the presence or absence of symptoms of a disease. It is like an on/off switch. If a genetic disease shows full penetrance, then every carrier of a gene mutation will show some symptom of the disease. If there are people who carry a mutation in a particular gene but show no symptoms of the disease, the disease is said to have reduced penetrance. An individual who carries a mutated gene but does not show symptoms of the disease is said to be nonpenetrant.

Reduced penetrance is generally more frequent with dominant diseases than with recessive diseases. For some genetic diseases, reduced penetrance is characteristic, but for other genetic diseases, carriers of gene mutations will always be symptomatic. For example, reduced penetrance is not generally believed to be a factor of achondroplasia. In other words, if you have the gene mutation, you have achondroplasia.

On the other hand, inherited forms of cancer frequently show reduced penetrance. For example, in families with inherited breast cancer, women that carry causative gene mutations may have a significantly greater risk, 80 to 90 percent in some cases, of developing breast cancer at some point in their lives, but it is not necessarily guaranteed that every gene carrier must develop breast cancer. Usually, the relative penetrance of the disease increases with the age of the at-risk individual, but it may never reach 100 percent.

"Variability" is a term used to describe the variety of different symptoms that can be seen in carriers of mutations in a given gene. It is like a volume adjustment. Many genetic diseases can cause a variety of symptoms in affected individuals, but not all symptoms may be present in all affected individuals. For example, some patients may show a particular symptom or set of symptoms, while others may show a different symptom or symptoms. Symptoms may also vary from mild to severe. Age of onset of the disease can vary as well. The reasons for variations in symptoms in carriers of the same gene mutation are not known but are probably due to additional genetic and/or environmental influences interacting with the disease genes.

Marfan syndrome is an example of a highly variable disorder. In Marfan syndrome, 30 to 60 percent of patients have scoliosis, 50 to 80 percent of patients have dislocation of the lenses of the eye, about 50 percent of children and 80 percent of adults have dilation of the aorta, and about 70 percent have mitral valve prolapse. Clearly, a majority but not necessarily all Marfan syndrome patients exhibit each of these symptoms, making the precise collection of symptoms and the severity of the disease variable from individual to individual.

Reduced penetrance and variability may sometimes make a genetic disease appear to skip a generation. If a particular individual in a family is either nonpenetrant or very mildly affected, it may appear that they are not a carrier of the gene when in fact they are. In such cases, individuals can carry a gene mutation that is clinically unrecognized. The uncertainties of penetrance and variability can also complicate the diagnosis of genetic disease because it may be difficult to determine if a disease was in fact inherited from a parent or occurred as a new mutation. Finally, the uncertainties of penetrance and variability can complicate the prediction of the disease risk in children. Genetic or other types of medical testing, if available, may clarify the situation for patients and families.

Diagnosis of highly variable genetic diseases can be made more difficult by uncharacteristic presentations of symptoms in some patients. For example, if a genetic disease shares symptoms with other diseases, it can be difficult to determine which one of a set of candidate diseases the person actually has. Accurate diagnosis is necessary if doctors are to provide good estimates of prognosis, risk for other family members, and the effectiveness of treatments. Genetic testing, when available, can be a precise tool for clarifying a clinical diagnosis. This option will be discussed in greater detail in Chapters 16, 17, and 18.

In addition, individuals in very large families or in families that live in different cities or countries may lose touch with each other, and important information regarding the health and physical characteristics of distant relatives can be lost. Because the patient may not be aware of potentially affected relatives, or because those relatives may be unavailable for clinical evaluation, it can sometimes be more difficult to diagnose a genetic condition with reduced penetrance or high variability. For this reason, it is important to provide your physician with as much family history information as possible when answering questions about the possibility of genetic disease, even if some of it seems inconsequential.

Genetic Heterogeneity

There are two types of genetic heterogeneity. One is called "allelic heterogeneity." Allelic heterogeneity occurs when a genetic disease is caused by different mutations in the same gene. This means that, while all patients with a particular disease have mutations in the same gene, they may not all have identical changes in the DNA sequence of that gene.

For example, cystic fibrosis (CF) is a genetic disease that shows allelic heterogeneity. CF is inherited in an autosomal recessive manner and is due to mutations in the cystic fibrosis gene—called the "cystic fibrosis transmembrane conductance regulator" or CFTR. The gene that causes CF is located on chromosome 7, an autosomal chromosome. Mutations in the CFTR gene interfere with the ability of cells to transport certain molecules—particularly chloride—across their cell membranes. The defect in cellular function is noted primarily in pancreatic, lung, genital, and sweat gland cells. Mutations in the CFTR gene cause symptoms that can include chronic obstructive lung disease and pancreatic insufficiency. Patients with CF have mutations in both of their CFTR genes on each of their chromosome 7s.

Despite the fact that all CF patients have mutations in the CFTR gene, those patients can carry a variety of different genetic alterations with the CFTR gene. As such, CF shows allelic heterogeneity. This is because, while CF may not always be caused by the exact same DNA mutation, it is always due to mutations in the same gene and is always inherited as an autosomal recessive disorder.

Sometimes, a genetic disease can be caused by mutations in any one of a number of different genes. This is called "locus heterogeneity" because mutations in different genes—or different genetic loci—can result in the same medical condition. Genetic diseases that show locus heterogeneity can demonstrate either a single pattern of inheritance or a number of different patterns of inheritance.

One disease that shows locus heterogeneity is hereditary nonpolyposis colon cancer or HNPCC. HNPCC is inherited in an autosomal dominant manner but can be due to mutations in any one of at least five different genes. The five genes that have been identified so far to be responsible for HNPCC include genes located on autosomal chromosomes 2, 3, and 7. The proteins made by these genes help to repair mismatches in base pairing of DNA nucleotides. The failure of DNA mismatch repair results in the accumulation of errors in the DNA message after repeated mitoses. Cells that show this defect are called "replication error positive," or RER+. The accumulation of errors in DNA results in the development of a heritable form of colon cancer. It is likely that these genes are also often involved in many cases of nonhereditary or sporadic colon cancer.

HNPCC shows locus heterogeneity because it can be caused by mutations in any one of several different genes. HNPCC can also show allelic heterogeneity because not all patients with mutations in a particular gene will necessarily have exactly the same genetic defect. However, despite the number of genes capable of causing the physical symptoms of colon cancer, the disease still follows an autosomal dominant pattern of inheritance. In this case, the importance of genetic heterogeneity is that it may be necessary to determine the specific gene at fault in any particular family in order to accurately determine the risk of the disease occurring in children and other relatives of the patient.

Consider a family that has HNPCC due to a mutation in the gene on chromosome 2. For this family, there is no reason to try to trace the inheritance of the chromosome 3 or 7 genes by relatives. Studying the inheritance of the chromosome 2 gene in the family will be all that is necessary for genetic diagnosis and assessment of disease risk. Studying the chromosome 3 and 7 genes in this case will not provide useful information.

Alternatively, retinitis pigmentosa (RP) can be inherited in an autosomal dominant, autosomal recessive, or X-linked manner, and can be due to mutations in several different genes. RP is characterized by degeneration of the retina of the eye leading to visual impairment and blindness. Genes responsible for RP have been localized to several different autosomal chromosomes as well as the X chromosome. RP can also be observed in association with other genetic syndromes. The genetic heterogeneity of RP lies not only in the variety of genes and mutations that can cause the disease, but also in the variety of ways that RP can be inherited and transmitted from generation to generation. Genetic testing, where available, and analysis of family history will be crucial to any estimation of how RP is being passed through a family.

The different patterns of inheritance observed with diseases showing locus heterogeneity are usually due to the differing effects of mutations in different genes. Imagine if there are several proteins that act together or as steps in a pathway to complete a certain task. Mutations in the gene for any particular protein in the pathway could cause similar clinical symptoms because of disruption of the entire pathway. However, mutations in the different genes may be inherited and manifested in different ways depending on the gene, its function in the pathway, and its chromosomal location.

HNPCC and RP are not the only diseases that show locus heterogeneity. Although the symptoms of such heterogeneous diseases may be fairly consistent regardless of which gene carries mutations, the implications for risk in other family members and children can be profound.

Genetic counseling for diseases showing locus heterogeneity will sometimes involve medical assessment of the patient and several relatives, information gathering about family history and ethnic background, and genetic testing, if available. All of the information that can be learned about a patient and his or her family may be required for doctors and genetic counselors to be able to determine the pattern of inheritance of the disease in the patient and estimate the possibility that other family members or children may be at risk. In such circumstances, patients may occasionally be asked about the availability or willingness of relatives to participate in genetic testing procedures.

Imprinting

Some genetic diseases only occur if a mutation is inherited from a particular parent, either the mother or the father. This is due to a process called "imprinting," which has only recently been explained. Imprinting in genetic disease is seen because, even though we each have two copies of autosomal genes (one gene on each chromosome of a pair), the two genes may not both be expressed (or made into RNA) at equal levels. Some genes are expressed only from the gene on the chromosome inherited from the father and not from the gene inherited from the mother. For other genes, the opposite may be true. Not all genes in the human genome are imprinted. But genes that show unequal levels of transcription from the two alleles are being discovered rapidly as we learn more about the imprinted regions of human chromosomes.

Imagine a gene that is expressed from the chromosome inherited from your mother and not from your father. If you inherit a mutation in that gene from your mother, you would be at risk for the disease because your cells will try to use that gene. Inheriting the mutant gene from your father, however, would not cause disease because your father's gene is not used.

Alternatively, if a gene is expressed only from your father's chromosome and not from your mother's, the only way to have disease symptoms would be to inherit a mutation from your father. Inheriting a mutation from your mother should not pose a problem.

Consider a female patient with a genetic disease caused because she inherited a mutation from her father in a gene expressed only from her father's chromosome. The gene inherited from her mother is silent. If the gene is only expressed from the father's chromosome, she could pass the mutation to her children, but they would not show symptoms of the disease because they would inherit the mutation from her, their mother. It is the children's father's gene, which is presumably not altered, that would be used. However, if this woman passes the mutation to a son, he could be at risk for passing the mutation and the disease to his children, even thought he is not affected by the disease. Also, any unaffected daughters could, through their sons, pass the disease to future generations. In such circumstances, the disease might appear to skip a generation or more.

Imprinting can also be a factor when, because of errors in cell division, both chromosomes of a pair are inherited from a single parent and no chromosome is inherited from the other parent. This phenomenon is called "uniparental disomy," or UPD. Imagine, for example, that there was a gene that was not expressed from the father's chromosome 15 and only expressed from the mother's chromosome 15. What would happen if, due to an error in mitosis or meiosis, a child carried two chromosome 15s from the father and no chromosome 15 from the mother? There would be a failure to express the gene in question because no source for the expression of the gene would exist.

Prader-Willi syndrome (PWS) is an example of an imprinted genetic disease that is caused when certain mutations occur on the chromosome 15 inherited from the father. Angelman syndrome (AS) is caused by certain mutations occurring on the chromosome 15 inherited from the mother. The genes involved in PWS and AS lie very close to each other in the same region of chromosome 15. PWS and AS can also be cause by UPD for chromosome 15.

We are only beginning to understand the importance of imprinting in genetic disease and to learn which genes in humans are imprinted. Future research will undoubtedly provide a great deal more information and help us understand the causes of many currently confusing genetic diseases.

Somatic Mosaicism

There are some genetic diseases that are the result of mutations that occur during the growth and development of an individual. In these cases, the fertilized egg did not carry the mutation and the mutation was not inherited from a parent. Instead, the mutation occurred in a cell, sometime during the cell divisions of growth and development. "Somatic mutation" diseases will appear as sporadic or new mutation diseases. Just like sporadic or new mutation genetic diseases, somatic diseases are genetic because they are caused by alterations in genes, but they are not inherited because the mutation did not come from a parent. Somatic mutations are carried by some but not all of the cells of an individual. As such, that individual is said to have somatic mosaicism.

Somatic mutations occur in somatic cells. Somatic cells are the cells of the body produced in mitosis during growth and development. Somatic cells are different from germ cells, which are cells that are destined to become sperm or egg cells.

Somatic mutations occur because of errors in duplication of the genome or after DNA damage. Somatic mutations are probably reasonably frequent, but if only a few cells are affected, the mutations may not have much of an effect on the individual. Since many somatic mutations may not cause a physical effect on a person, they are likely to go unnoticed, and estimates of how frequently they really occur are only obtained through research. Somatic mutations will result in genetic disease only when they are present in enough cells or when they disrupt a critical protein in a certain subset of cells.

True somatic mutations are not passed to future generations because they do not involve germ cells. In some cases, it may be difficult to determine whether the germ cells of the affected individual also carry the new mutation, which would indicate gonadal mosaicism in addition to somatic mosaicism. If the germ cells of the affected individual also carry the mutation, then there is a risk of passing the mutation to a future generation.

A classic example of somatic mutations that result in genetic disease is cancer. In cancer, some cells of an individual acquire somatic mutations that disrupt the control of cell division. These mutations cause uncontrolled growth of a set of cells. Cancer mutations and their impact on an individual is discussed in more detail in the next chapter.

Multifactorial Inheritance

"Multifactorial inheritance" is a pattern of inheritance characterized by the contribution of multiple factors, genetic and nongenetic, to the occurrence of a disease. In multifactorial diseases, more than one gene may be involved in the appearance of a trait or condition, and some variable number of environmental factors is also required. As such, the causes of multifactorial diseases can be difficult to characterize because of the variety of genetic and environmental factors that must all be present.

Many human disorders such as hypertension, insulin dependent diabetes, multiple sclerosis, and obesity are considered multifactorial with major genetic components that act in combination with environmental influences. Until all the genetic and nongenetic influences are sorted out, causes may sometimes appear to differ from patient to patient.

Apparent differences in causation can also complicate research, diagnosis, and treatment. Sorting out which genetic and environmental factors are crucial to development of a disease and which are not is very difficult. The ambiguities can make clarification of the causes of a disease a complicated undertaking. Family studies are important for research on multifactorial diseases because of the genetic elements that are shared by the members of a family. Epidemiologic studies are also important because they help to identify common environmental influences present in the geographical areas where the disease is most common.

Genetic research is teaching us about many of the different genetic and environmental influences involved in these and other complicated diseases. Determining which genetic influences are at work is important to developing useful genetic tests for multifactorial diseases. Understanding the genetics is also important for estimating genetic risk for other members of a family.

Determining the environmental influences that contribute to the development of a multifactorial disease is important because knowing the environmental factors involved can lead to the development of prevention strategies. Prevention might, in some cases, be as simple as avoidance of contributing factors by individuals with genetic risk factors. For example, while we still do not know all of the contributing factors for heart disease we have learned enough so that doctors often suggest certain types of diets or medications for patients with particular risk factors such as high blood pressure or high cholesterol.

For many multifactorial diseases, we still do not know enough about the causes to give patients a good explanation of why the disease occurred, but the ability to provide risk estimates to relatives is becoming more accurate because of research. In the future, personalized diagnosis and treatment methods may be available for many multifactorial diseases. For example, there are many genetic and nongenetic factors that contribute to traits such as blood pressure levels. Not all factors may be at work in all patients with high blood pressure. Understanding the individual genetic factors at work in each particular case might allow a physician to choose among different treatment options and customize treatments to each patient's individual needs. Customized treatments are potentially much more effective than generalized ones because they would go directly to the cause of each patient's symptoms.

In Conclusion

Because of the complexities of imprinting, somatic mutation, gonadal mosaicism, genetic heterogeneity, penetrance and variability, anticipation, and multifactorial inheritance, it is important for patients and families with concerns about genetically influenced disease to seek professional genetic counseling and clinical genetics care. Geneticists can help patients obtain diagnostic confirmation, identify the possible factors at work in their particular cases, learn about future risks for themselves and their families, and explore what additional medical assistance may be available.

CHAPTER TWELVE

Nonhereditary and Nongenetic Disease

As we learned in the previous chapter, some diseases, while not inherited from one's parents, may still be genetic. Even though not inherited, these types of genetic disease are still the result of alterations in the genetic information of the affected individual. This type of genetic disease applies in particular to sporadic or new mutation genetic diseases or somatic mosaicism, as described in the previous chapter.

Nonhereditary Disease

We already know that sporadic or nonhereditary genetic diseases can be caused by mutations that occurred in genes during DNA replication, mitosis, or meiosis. Sometimes, however, sporadic genetic diseases can be caused by "mutagens." Mutagens are substances that cause DNA damage and induce mutations. Mutagenic substances include many chemicals and radiation. Mutagens can be naturally occurring or man-made substances. Not all substances encountered or made by man are mutagenic.

Induced DNA mutations can cause a variety of medical problems depending upon when the exposure to the mutagen occurred, how much of the mutagen was encountered, and which cells may have been damaged. For example, exposure to small amounts of a mutagen late in life is likely to affect only a small number of cells. Damage to the genes of a small number of cells may never result in observable physical effects. However, just because an exposure to a mutagen may be quite limited or occur late in development does not necessarily mean it is safe.

On the other hand, a large-dose exposure to a mutagen, especially in an embryo or small child, may result in DNA damage to a significant proportion of cells. Exposures to many cells, exposures early in development, or long-term exposures to a mutagen may cause significant medical problems. Furthermore, any exposure to a mutagen can be devastating if it causes the wrong type of DNA damage. The most visible example of a disease caused by exposure to a mutagen is cancer.

Cancer is observed as the uncontrolled mitosis of cells in the body. Scientists now know that there are many genes within cells that tightly regulate the rate and timing of mitosis. Some genes encourage cells to divide, while some genes do exactly the opposite and inhibit or slow cell division. These genes work together in a well-balanced, carefully choreographed way to keep the cells of the body in check.

In cancer, cells lose the ability to regulate mitosis, causing unregulated division of cells. Cancer-causing mutations can be the result of improperly functioning DNA replication machinery, errors that randomly occur during copying of the genetic information, or exposure to mutagens. Prolonged exposure to mutagens can overwhelm the DNA repair processes, speed the appearance of multiple mutations, and accelerate the progression of a cell to a cancerous state.

During the development of cancer, genes that slow mitosis are inactivated or switched off. Concurrently, genes that encourage cell division are permanently activated or switched on. The combination of these mutations causes a cell to lose control of mitosis. Except for familial cancer syndromes where the pathway toward cancer is initiated by mutations inherited from a parent, cancer-causing mutations are generally somatic in nature and occur during the lifetime of the affected individual. It is now thought that cancer develops as a step-by-step process wherein a number of mutations must occur over time, and mutations must occur in many different genes. Since mutations in many genes are required for cancer to develop, the process is generally considered to be a gradual progression in a cell from a controlled, noncancerous state to a malignant, cancerous state.

Many genes have been discovered that help control cell division. Certain mutations in specific genes can be found in a variety of types of tumors throughout the body. For example, mutations in a gene called p53 are commonly found in tumors of many different origins. On the other hand, mutations in some other genes are more likely to be specific to a particular type of tumor. Recent research has identified specific gene mutations characteristic to breast and ovarian tumors or tumors of the colon, lung, or prostate.

With respect to cancer induced by exposure to mutagens, different mutagens may be more likely to induce a particular type of cancer based on the site of exposure and mode of action. For example, exposure to ultraviolet rays from the sun is more likely to cause skin cancer than other types of cancer, while smoking is more likely to cause lung cancer, and chewing tobacco is more likely to cause mouth, esophageal, and stomach cancer.

Genetic research geared toward identifying the genes involved in cancer and understanding the mutations that play a role in cancer is important because it points to possible new methods of diagnosis and treatment. For example, if certain types of tumors are found to frequently carry mutations in specific genes, individuals can be tested for mutations in those genes to assess their risk for developing that particular type of tumor.

Research focused on identifying the early, precancerous genetic changes characteristic of many types of tumors, such as breast, lung and prostate tumors, may provide for early detection of a person's susceptibility to develop cancer. Imagine how powerful it could be to screen for the early genetic changes that lead to the development of prostate cancer. Genetic testing could be used to detect these early changes, before the progression to cancer is complete. Early detection can lead to early intervention. Early intervention could be curative. The hope is that treating patients before the appearance of outward symptoms and spread of disease will result in improved survival for many types of cancer.

Genetic research may also one day suggest new treatment approaches for cancer. In conventional treatments such as surgery or radiation, the idea is to remove or destroy the cancerous tissue and thereby remove or kill the cells carrying cancerous mutations. However, if mutant cells remain, there will be a risk for recurrence of the tumor in the patient. If an understanding is developed of the genes that cause the problem, then treatment methods such as drugs or gene therapy might be designed that can efficiently target cancer cells throughout the body and either help cells regain control of cell division or systematically destroy the cancer cells. Such treatments would be designed to interfere with the function of the altered proteins and stop the uncontrolled cell division. Effective drug or gene therapy treatments may one day provide nonsurgical approaches to stopping tumor growth. These types of treatments have the potential to reduce the risk of tumor recurrence by efficiently destroying cancer cells, wherever they reside in the body. Such approaches may also provide new options for patients with inoperable tumors or advanced metastatic disease.

In addition to its diagnostic capabilities, genetic testing in cancer has a variety of potential research applications because there are many things left to learn about how cancer affects the body. Sensitive, specific genetic tests provide a tool for answering a number of questions. First, DNA mutations can be compared among tumors located throughout the body. Identifying the genetic mutations carried by tumors at different places in the body can help doctors study mechanisms of metastasis.

Genetic tests also provide a powerful tool for identifying one cell that carries a genetic defect out of a huge number of cells that do not. Such studies may be useful for assessing the effectiveness of treatments by detecting small numbers of cancer cells that have survived treatments such as chemotherapy, surgery, or gene therapy. Finally, genetic tests might be used to characterize the mutations present in a patient's tissues. Characterizing the precise mutations present in different types of tumors has been shown to be useful in diagnosing cancers, estimating the prognosis for the patient, and predicting the aggressiveness of the tumor. In the future, different treatments for many cancers may be specifically developed for particular genetic mutations.

Nongenetic Disease

Although the subject of this book is hereditary genetic disease and its complications, we must remember that people are frequently afflicted with disorders that have no genetic basis. For example, bacterial and viral infections are clearly acquired diseases that are not genetic and are not necessarily transmitted from one's parents. Other examples include broken bones and other types of injuries, wounds, or trauma. Without some underlying reason for frequent recurrence of nongenetic disease, such as a genetic basis for immunodeficiency that results in recurrent infections or a genetic basis for fragile bones such as mild osteogenesis imperfecta, many medical problems are not necessarily related to genetics.

Another cause of human illness that is often seen by geneticists is that of birth defects caused by fetal exposure to harmful substances. "Teratogens" are the classic examples. Teratogens are substances that cause abnormalities in fetuses and newborns that are not due to mutations in genes.

Many different substances have the potential to exert damaging effects on fetuses. Some substances are known to be safe while others are known to be dangerous. Dangerous substances can include certain legal and illegal drugs or medications, alcohol, chemicals, viruses, and bacteria. The damaging effects of teratogens depend upon many factors including the method and site of action of the substance, the time during pregnancy at which exposure occurs, the duration of the exposure, and the dosage.

One frequently reported teratogen is alcohol. Alcohol use during pregnancy can cause certain birth defects or abnormalities in a child that are not likely to occur without the use of alcohol by the mother. In addition, many drugs such as some kinds of antidepressants, anticonvulsants, and antibiotics can cause certain characteristic fetal abnormalities. Some drugs carry presently unknown risks.

Some parasitic, bacterial, and viral exposures should also be avoided by pregnant women whenever possible. One example is toxoplasmosis. Toxoplasma gondii is a parasite frequently found in cat feces. Exposure of pregnant women to the toxoplasma parasite has received quite a bit of public attention recently because of the potential for birth defects. As a result, it is gen-erally recommended that pregnant women avoid contact with used cat litter.

Because of the potential for fetal abnormalities due to infectious agents or drug use during pregnancy, women who are pregnant or planning a preg-nancy should consult with their physicians about the risk of birth defects from parasites, bacteria, viruses, or any substances or drugs to which the fetus might be exposed. In addition, women should make sure that their doctors are aware of the medications they take and ask about the teratogenic potential and appropriate doses of such medications during pregnancy.

In contrast to teratogens, there are a few substances that have been determined to be beneficial. For example, it is now recommended that all women of childbearing age ingest at least 0.4 milligrams of supplemental folic acid each day. Adequate intake of folic acid has been shown to reduce the incidence of neural-tube defects in children.

As our understanding of human genes improves, scientists are learning about the many genetic factors that modulate how our bodies respond to environmental influences such as mutagens and teratogens. Recent studies have shown that sometimes genes play a role in how our bodies respond to and process some chemicals and drugs. For example, some people metabo-lize isoniazid, a common drug used to treat tuberculosis, faster than others. As a result, dosages of some drugs may need to be adjusted to avoid unwanted side effects due to higher than needed doses in some patients and lack of effectiveness due to lower than needed doses in others.

It would not be surprising to find that some fetuses are more at risk for birth defects or serious side effects from many substances because of under-lying genetic factors in the mother and child. Unfortunately, tests or pre-ventive measures for most such genetic susceptibilities are likely to be far in the future. At present, the best course of action is avoidance, where pos-sible, of substances known to be harmful.

One additional area of genetic research that is receiving a great deal of attention is the focus on identifying the genetic basis of susceptibility to infec-tious agents such as viruses. We are learning that some people are more natu-rally susceptible to certain infectious agents, while some people appear more naturally resistant. For example, recent evidence has shown that there is a genetic basis for resistance to infection by the human immunodeficiency virus, HIV. It would not be surprising to learn that this is not the only such example. A number of genetic factors may influence our susceptibility to many infectious agents. Future research will likely teach us why some individuals are more naturally resistant to certain infectious agents, and may provide clues about how to treat or even prevent illness in susceptible individuals.

CHAPTER THIRTEEN

When to Consider a Genetic Test

Medical tests are nothing new. Every one of us is likely to have some kind of medical test at one time or another during our lives. Doctors draw blood and take X-rays routinely. And like X-rays for seeing broken bones and blood tests for determining cell counts or cholesterol levels, there are now tests for studying the genes inside human cells.

Despite the routine nature of most other medical testing, genetic tests are considered by many people to be much more invasive. The genetic information derived from DNA testing is commonly thought to be potentially more dangerous than other types of medical information. Much like the concern for privacy in HIV testing, the fear of many people is that their genetic information might be misused in a variety of circumstances—especially if it is predictive of a possible future illness by which the individual is not currently affected.

Even though there may be many medical advantages for considering a genetic test, there may also be compelling social, legal, or personal reasons for not taking a genetic test. This chapter will focus on the medical aspects of genetic testing. Ethical, social, legal, and other common concerns about genetic testing will be addressed in the next chapter.

From a purely medical standpoint, individuals may choose to have a genetic test in any of the following situations.

Genetic tests can confirm a diagnosis made by a doctor during clinical examination of a patient. In cases where a patient presents with symptoms that are suggestive of any one of a number of possible diseases, a genetic test, if available, may help the doctor refine and clarify a diagnosis. The confirmation of a diagnosis of genetic disease can be important for prognosis, treatment, and estimating risk for the disease in other family members and future generations.

Genetic tests can be used to diagnose individuals with atypical disease—that is, nonpenetrant disease, highly variable symptoms, or very mild presentation. For example, if a patient has a relative with a particular genetic disease and the patient's own medical status is unclear, or if a patient has symptoms consistent with some aspects of a disease but not enough symptoms for a firm diagnosis, a genetic test can answer many questions. Such diagnostic information may be important for developing the best course of treatment for the patient and for estimating disease risk for relatives and children.

In cases where there is a family history of recessive genetic disease, genetic tests can be used to identify unaffected carriers and carrier couples where both partners are unaffected carriers. Unaffected carriers of recessive genetic diseases, while generally asymptomatic themselves, can have an increased risk of having affected children if their partners are also carriers. In these cases, determination of a person's carrier status can provide more accurate estimates of disease risk in children than would be possible without genetic testing.

Genetic tests can identify unaffected carriers of recessive genetic diseases who do not have a family history of the disease. Programs called "carrier screening" programs are conducted for large numbers of individuals without regard to family history. Widespread carrier screening programs can have an impact on disease incidence, particularly in populations with a greatly increased incidence of a particular recessive disease. An example of a recessive genetic disease with variable risk among different populations is Tay-Sachs disease. Individuals of Ashkenazi Jewish descent have a greater risk than non-Jewish individuals of being carriers of Tay-Sachs disease and of having children with the disease. In such populations, organized carrier screening in conjunction with education and genetic counseling can be of great benefit to couples planning families. However, generalized carrier screening for genetic disease may not always be beneficial, especially in the absence of good public education about genetic disease. As certain genetic tests with widespread screening capabilities become available, it will be important for society to weigh the benefits, limitations, and risks before considering large-scale implementation of screening programs.

Genetic tests can be used to identify individuals at risk for future disease who are not currently symptomatic. This capability represents perhaps the most feared potential of genetic testing. For readily treatable adult onset diseases such as inherited colon or breast cancer, determination of who in a family is at risk for future disease may allow physicians to provide better monitoring and treatment, thereby improving survival and quality of life. In families such as this, genetic tests can also identify individuals who are not at increased risk and release them from anxiety, unnecessary further testing, and additional expense. Guaranteed confidentiality of test results is important for this application of genetic testing so that patients can trust that their genetic information will not be misused and that they will not be discriminated against because of the test results.

On the other hand, presymptomatic genetic testing for untreatable diseases such as Huntington disease can be highly controversial because, without effective treatment, genetic test results can have profound psychological and social effects on patients and their families. Genetic counseling, confidentiality of test results, and the freedom of patients to make their own decisions about whether or not to be tested are an important part of testing in these cases.

Genetic tests can detect genetic diseases prenatally. Prenatal genetic testing is now available for a number of genetic conditions, including Down syndrome, Turner syndrome, trisomy 13, trisomy 18, Klinefelter syndrome, cystic fibrosis, Tay-Sachs disease, Gaucher disease, achondroplasia, Duchenne muscular dystrophy, alpha-1 antitrypsin deficiency, hemophilia, myotonic dystrophy, sickle cell disease, and many, many others.

It is becoming increasingly common for expectant parents to use genetic testing to assess the genetic health of their children. Expectant parents who have a family history of a particular genetic disease often use genetic tests to determine whether or not their child is at risk for the disease. Expectant parents also frequently use genetic testing to assess the number of chromosomes in the fetus to determine whether their baby carries an aneuploidy. For example, pregnant women who are concerned about Down syndrome in their unborn child can have prenatal genetic testing performed to determine the number of chromosome 21s carried by the child. Prenatal testing can also determine the sex of the fetus.

How Genetic Testing Is Performed

Genetic testing is performed on DNA isolated from the cells of the individual undergoing testing. A variety of tissues can provide cells from which DNA can be isolated. The tissue sample needed generally depends upon the disease in question and the testing methods being used.

In children and adults, the most common procedure for collecting cells for genetic tests is to draw blood, usually by needle from the arm. The white blood cells called lymphocytes are purified from the rest of the blood components. DNA is extracted from lymphocytes for examination of chromosomes or genes. With some of the newer technologies, a drop of blood from a finger stick or a sample of cells (called buccal cells) swabbed from the inside of the cheek may be all that is necessary. The advantages of these cell extraction methods is that they are less invasive and less painful, but they also yield many fewer cells and far less DNA. As such, these methods may not provide enough DNA for some procedures.

Sometimes DNA tests are not necessary for diagnosing a genetic disease. For example, sometimes a blood or urine sample can be used to diagnose a genetic disease through biochemical analysis of blood or urine content.

Occasionally, a tissue biopsy is needed to study a gene from a particular tissue. In these cases, a sample is removed from an appropriate tissue or organ. The method for obtaining the tissue sample will vary depending upon the location within the body of the sample required. For example, in cancer where tumor cells may carry a genetic mutation not found in other cells, a tissue biopsy of the tumor may be necessary for relevant DNA testing.

In prenatal genetic studies, fetal cells must be collected in order to examine the DNA from the child. Currently, methods such as "amniocentesis," "chorionic villus sampling," or "cordocentesis" are used to obtain fetal cells for analysis.

In amniocentesis, fetal cells contained within the amniotic fluid are extracted by transabdominal needle aspiration of amniotic fluid. Amniocentesis is
typically performed at around sixteen to eighteen weeks of pregnancy.

The DNA isolated from amniotic cells can be used in a variety of genetic tests. Other analyses such as measurement of enzyme activities or detection of biochemical compounds can also be performed on amniotic fluid
samples. Certain enzymatic or biochemical anomalies can be indicative of
genetic diseases. For example, detection of atypical levels of alpha-fetoprotein in amniotic fluid can be suggestive of many problems, including incor-
rect estimation of due date, twin pregnancies, or fetal abnormalities such as
neural tube defects or Down syndrome. Alpha-fetoprotein levels can also be
measured from maternal blood serum, and in some cases this may be prefer-
able to amniocentesis. Although amniocentesis is performed fairly commonly today by many doctors, it is an invasive procedure and does carry a
small but measurable risk for the fetus.

In the procedure called chorionic villus sampling, or CVS, cells from the
chorionic villus, a tissue that surrounds the fetus, are extracted by needle
aspiration either transabdominally or transcervically. DNA isolated from
CVS tissue can be used in a variety of genetic tests. In addition, the samples can be analyzed for enzyme activities or protein or metabolite levels for
the detection of biochemical or metabolic anomalies. Testing of CVS tissue
is similar to the testing of amniocentesis samples, as described above.
However, one advantage of CVS is that it can be performed much earlier
than amniocentesis, typically at around nine to twelve weeks of pregnancy.
Although CVS is useful in many circumstances, CVS is an invasive medical procedure and carries a small but measurable risk for the fetus.

In cordocentesis, also called fetal blood sampling (FBS), fetal blood is
drawn by inserting a needle directly into the umbilical cord. DNA can be
extracted from the fetal blood lymphocytes for genetic testing. Fetal blood
can also be analyzed, just as with amniocentesis and CVS, for biochemical
composition. Chemical analyses on cordocentesis samples, such as measurement of enzyme activities or characterization of biochemical content,
can help to detect certain fetal anomalies. Like amniocentesis and CVS,

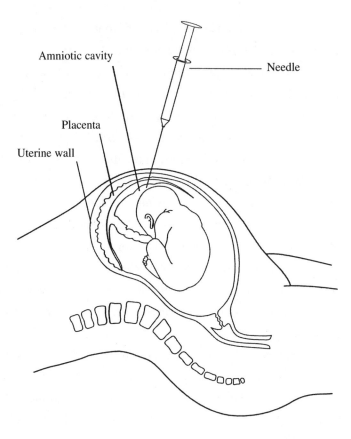

FIGURE 13.1 Diagram showing the transabdominal needle aspiration of amniotic fluid. Amniotic fluid and the cells contained in it can be used for genetic and biochemical assessment of a fetus.

cordocentesis is an invasive procedure that carries a small but measurable risk for the fetus.

Fetal cells and DNA obtained through amniocentesis, CVS, or cordocentesis can be examined directly or cultured and examined later, depending upon the requirements of the tests being performed. Each of these procedures for prenatal genetic testing can be very powerful, but each also has its limitations. For example, a normal test result does not always guarantee a normal child. Tests can only address the one condition for which they are designed.

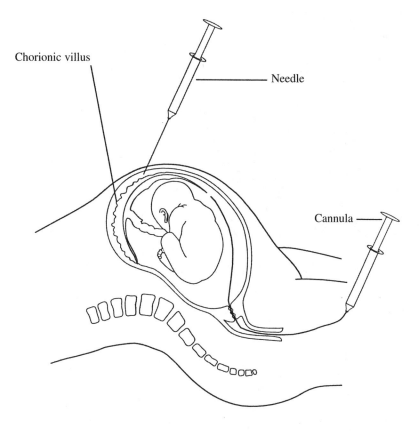

Chorionic villus

Needle

Cannula

FIGURE 13.2 Diagram showing the transabdominal and transcervical needle aspiration of chorionic villus samples. Chorionic villus tissue can be used for genetic and biochemical assessment of a fetus.

It is vitally important that the correct test be ordered because the right answers can only be obtained if the right questions are asked. For example, if one is concerned about Down syndrome in the pregnancy of a woman at age 38, cytogenetic analysis of fetal cells to count chromosomes is currently the most accurate way to ask about the chromosomal status of the fetus. However, a normal chromosome result from such an analysis cannot guarantee a completely healthy child and will not address whether the fetus will or will not have a single gene disorder such as CF.

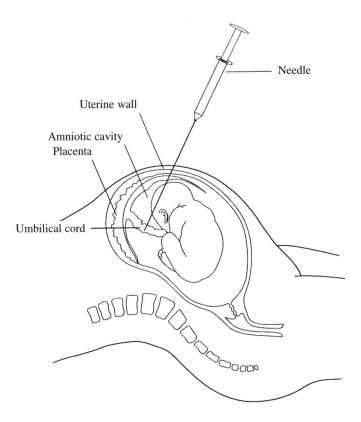

Needle

Uterine wall

Amniotic cavity
Placenta

Umbilical cord

FIGURE 13.3 Diagram showing the transabdominal collection of fetal blood cells by cordocentesis. Fetal blood can be used for genetic and biochemical assessment of a fetus.

Alternatively, a single gene test for CF in a child with a family history cannot address whether that child might also have another single gene disorder such as muscular dystrophy or a chromosomal disorder such as Down syndrome. This is because different genetic diseases involve different genes and/or chromosomes.

Separate tests would have to be ordered to assess the individual risk of each of these and other genetic conditions. However, separate tests may not always require separate samplings. For example, a single amniocentesis procedure often provides enough material for several genetic and biochemical tests, if the tests are all planned and a sufficient sample is collected.

Tests can only be effective and useful when used with a full understanding of their capabilities and limitations. The precise test performed will depend upon the disease in question. Patients and doctors need to understand what tests are being requested and what the capabilities of those tests are.

Finally, prenatal procedures, while fairly common in today's medical practice, also carry a level of risk for the fetus. It is important to consider the level of risk associated with whichever test is being considered and decide whether the need to know and the benefits of knowing outweigh the potential risks to the mother and fetus. For example, amniocentesis for the cytogenetic detection of Down syndrome is generally recommended for women when the age-associated risk of having a child with Down syndrome exceeds the risk of miscarriage after amniocentesis.

Advanced technologies are currently under development where fetal cells might be isolated from a blood sample drawn from the arm of the mother. Such an approach, if ultimately proven to be effective, should greatly reduce the risk to the fetus of performing prenatal testing procedures because it would eliminate the need to sample through the uterus and into the fetal environment.

There are a number of other, noninvasive testing methods that, even thought they do not test DNA directly, have applications for certain genetic conditions. Prenatal ultrasound uses high-frequency sound waves directed into the abdomen through a transducer placed against the abdominal wall. Ultrasound can be used to obtain a picture of the fetus and its internal organs. Ultrasound is frequently used to detect structural defects such as heart defects, neural tube defects, skeletal defects, and growth or placental abnormalities. The identification of some abnormalities may be suggestive of certain genetic conditions. Ultrasound can also be used after birth to detect anomalies in internal organs of children or adults.

Other noninvasive methods for looking inside the body to detect abnormalities include X-ray, CT (computed tomography) scan, PET (positron emission tomography) scan, and MRI (magnetic resonance imaging). These are widely used to test for genetic and nongenetic conditions and may be called upon to gather diagnostic information in many different circumstances.

Remember, medical testing gives doctors a way to ask the body questions about what may be wrong. Depending on the genetic disease suspected, doctors and patients will need to make a choice about the correct questions to ask and the way to ask them. Doctors will need to determine the samples needed and who in the family to test. Every genetic test has strengths, limitations, and risks. The decision about the type of test to use in a particular case is generally dependent upon the diagnosis being considered or the concerns of the patient.

Individuals interested in prenatal procedures should consult at length with their physicians about the advantages, capabilities, limitations, benefits, risks, and potential outcomes of each procedure before deciding to have a test.

CHAPTER FOURTEEN

Legal, Social, and Ethical Implications of a Genetic Test

The potential contribution of genetic research to medicine is immense. The pace at which genetic research proceeds is leading us into the future rapidly. Because of the success of genetic research efforts, we as a society are soon going to have to answer a number of legal, social, and ethical questions about the acceptable and appropriate use of medical genetic capabilities. Many complex issues such as assurance of the confidentiality of genetic information and protection against genetic discrimination in insurance and employment are already here. And, as genetic research continues, these and other complicated issues are likely to demand resolution.

When considering a genetic test, it is important for individuals to weigh the advantages and implications of genetic testing before and during the procedures. To do this, patients must educate themselves about their choices and understand the benefits, limitations, and risks of genetic tests, and for that matter any medical procedure, so that they can make informed choices about their medical care.

Clinical geneticists and genetic counselors can generally offer advice on the advantages and implications of genetic testing for different diseases. They can also provide information on alternatives throughout the process. Consulting a genetics specialist may be necessary unless your doctor has had formal training in genetics and/or extensive experience with the disease about which you are concerned. The purpose of this chapter is to present a variety of situations in which ethical, social, and legal questions arise.

Legal Issues

There are often compelling medical reasons for individuals to choose to have a genetic test. For example, when someone is showing symptoms suggestive of a certain genetic disease, there is usually little concern about genetic testing of the patient for confirmation of the diagnosis. Since the genetic diagnosis is suspected even without the genetic test, the fears concerning privacy or the effect the information will have on the patient's insurance or employment is not likely to be so great because the patient is already sick and carries a tentative diagnosis.

The advantages to having the test could include clarification of the diagnosis, more precise estimation of prognosis, more accurate prediction of risk for family members, and improved medical management of patients and families. However, it is also important to remember that the diagnosis of a genetic disease, with or without a genetic test, can have social, emotional, and psychological consequences for individuals and their families. These consequences can range from anxiety to guilt to fear to depression, which may make additional forms of medical assistance or support for patients and families necessary.

More complex legal and ethical questions arise in cases where a genetic test can identify a predisposition to develop a disease later in life. The first situation we will discuss involves diseases for which some form of treatment exists, like colon or breast cancer. From a medical standpoint, it may be advantageous to detect and diagnose a risk for such a disease early. But in the wrong hands, this information can be very harmful.

Say, for example, that colon cancer runs in your family and you want to know, for whatever reason, your chance of developing colon cancer based on whether or not you carry the at-risk gene. The advantages for you, your family, and your doctor if you are at increased risk could include more diligent screening, earlier detection, improved management, and possibly even prevention. If you are not at increased risk, you could avoid unnecessary anxiety and further medical procedures.

But what if your insurance company wanted to know the results of the genetic test so they could cancel your policy or charge you higher premiums based on an increased chance that you might get sick? Or, what if your employer wanted to know the results to determine whether or not you would be a good candidate for promotion? Patients should ask their physicians whether the laws in their state assure the confidentiality of genetic information and protect against genetic discrimination in insurance or employment.

What if you decided not to be tested? Could your insurance company or employer force you to take a genetic test just because it is available? What would they do with the information? Would it affect your insurance or employment? Would genetic testing or the use of genetic information for nonmedical purposes ever be in the best interests of the patient?

Many people would argue that any nonmedical use of genetic information is unacceptable—especially if genetic information is used to stigmatize or discriminate against a patient or the patient's family. Many would also argue that genetic information should be private and confidential between a doctor and patient and that the confidentiality of genetic information must be protected.

In cases such as this one, presymptomatic testing may have significant medical benefit—if there are treatments available that can improve the longevity and quality of life of the at-risk individual. Genetic testing and intensive screening combined with early detection and aggressive intervention might be life saving. But what steps must we as a society take to protect the patient's right to take advantage of the latest medical technology for his or her own benefit without the fear of genetic discrimination or loss of privacy?

Currently, predisposition to cancer is the most visible application of this type of presymptomatic genetic test, but as treatments improve for other diseases such as heart disease, multiple sclerosis, Alzheimer's disease, and Huntington disease, many more people are likely to consider presymptomatic genetic testing.

Sometimes the choices about genetic testing are not so straightforward. Some individuals may have compelling personal reasons not to have a genetic test. For example, in the case of healthy individuals considering presymptomatic testing for untreatable diseases, the choices are often very complicated. Different people will make different decisions about whether or not to be tested. And similar decisions may be reached by different people for different reasons.

In the absence of effective prevention or treatment for a disease, the possible beneficial applications and uses of the information should be weighed against the potential psychological, emotional, and legal implications of the test results. Concerns over the possibility of discrimination in employment and insurance should be considered by patients. Patients should find out about the current status of their state's laws that protect against such forms of discrimination.

Patients should also examine the real benefits of knowing the information. How will the information help them? How will it help their families? What do they plan to do with the information? How will it impact their lifestyle or planning for the future?

Presymptomatic genetic testing procedures for untreatable diseases can frequently have a profound impact beyond the individual, carrying implications for siblings, other relatives, or future generations. The choice about whether or not to take such a genetic test can be difficult, and patients may have a difficult time trying to make up their own minds about what they want—especially if they feel pressure from others. The freedom of patients to make their own choices in such matters, without the intervention of others, is important. And avoidance of genetic discrimination by insurance companies and employers promises to be a topic of heated legal and social debate in coming years.

These are just two examples in which concerns about genetic testing can arise for patients. These examples alone raise questions such as how do we preserve the patient's and doctor's rights to voluntarily and appropriately take advantage of the medical genetic alternatives for patient care? How do we protect ourselves against misuse of genetic tests and information?

The misuse of genetic information is most often thought of in relation to social stigmatization or discrimination. Discrimination can come in the form of denial of life insurance, health insurance, or employment. Concerns over genetic discrimination raise questions about the confidentiality of medical records, including genetic test results.

In the United States, many states have already passed laws that protect against discrimination based on information from genetic tests. These laws are designed to prohibit the inappropriate use of genetic information. Many other states are considering such legislation. The federal government is also considering legislation written specifically to protect against genetic discrimination.

Until these laws are passed in all states or by the federal government, concerns about whether genetic information could be used against you by your insurers or employers are very real for some patients. It also may be unclear how such test results would impact you if you were to move to another state, change jobs, or apply to a new insurance company. Your genetic counselor, physician, or clinical geneticist may be able to provide up-to-date information about the laws in your state and how genetic test results might be protected. These professionals may also be able to provide or obtain information about which genetic tests insurance companies will pay for and which they will not.

Clearly, current legislation will need to be updated as scientific advances are made that render it inadequate or obsolete. Educated and thoughtful public input will be necessary and important in the development of laws that protect the rights of all individuals.

There are also important legal and medical issues to consider in the regulation of genetic tests. For example, even though a new test could potentially be informative and useful, there are frequently limitations, error rates, and social implications of the procedure to consider in light of the potential advance. This issue is confronted frequently by the medical community when trying to balance the potential importance of new procedures against the potential risks.

Most people would agree that potentially useful drugs and procedures, particularly those that can benefit patients with no other options or those that patients are demanding, should be brought to the public as quickly as possible. But a bad testing procedure, just like a drug with devastating side effects, may be very harmful. As a result, scientists ask whether the new method is as effective as it could be and whether the risks and limitations outweigh the potential benefits. As we have seen in recent years with possible new treatments for cancer and AIDS, such issues are often the source of great debate both among members of the medical community and between medical professionals and patients.

A recent example of the debate over widespread application of a genetic test centered around the ability to detect carriers for cystic fibrosis (CF) with high sensitivity and great accuracy. Given the accuracy and reliability of the new test, should widespread mandatory CF carrier testing be implemented?

Some people feel that population screening might have some use, but there are still many unanswered questions about the benefits and risks of such procedures—especially since there is currently no cure for the disease. The level of public education about genetic testing in general and about CF in particular is still fairly low. Universal implementation of the procedure has not been recommended because further studies are needed to assess how the information would be used, how it would affect individuals who were tested, and what medical and legal infrastructure needs to be provided to optimize the effectiveness of such testing. Carrier testing for CF is, however, currently available on demand to interested individuals and couples.

Alternatively, phenylketonuria (PKU), another autosomal recessive genetic disease, is routinely tested for at birth because treatment is simple and effective. Dietary management of phenylalanine intake can avoid the devastating effects of the disease. In this case, without question, the benefits far outweigh the risks.

Is the availability of curative treatment what tips the scale? Maybe. But when should screening move from being voluntary to being mandatory? And who pays for mandatory testing? What bearing does the frequency of the disease and cost to society of managing sick patients versus the cost of performing the test on a large scale have on the implementation of a screening program?

Social Issues

A variety of social issues arise from genetic testing situations. As previously discussed, the diagnosis of a genetic disease in a family can have significant psychological and emotional effects. For example, in the case of healthy individuals considering carrier screening for recessive diseases, either with or without a family history, the identification of a risk for passing a genetic disease to future generations can raise a number of questions about how to use the information and how to assess the risk for genetic disease in children. Carrier screening can impact other family members, especially if a disease gene is found that was previously unsuspected. Families can suddenly find themselves facing a number of difficult choices, including whether and how to use this information.

Other social issues can include lost information in families where relatives are unavailable or unwilling to participate in genetic studies. In most cases, this becomes an issue only when relatives are needed for diagnosis or to trace the inheritance of a disease gene in a family. Balancing the right to know of individuals who desire testing against the rights of individuals who do not can be challenging. These and other social issues can be discussed with your physician or genetic counselor prior to, during, and after genetic testing. Careful consideration of the issues can help families make decisions about the management of genetic information.

Ethical Issues

Many people believe that patients and families should be educated and informed about genetic tests that are being offered and should provide statements assuring their informed consent to and voluntary participation in the procedures. However, this can sometimes be a complex issue. For example, if an individual is exhibiting symptoms characteristic of a particular genetic disease, is genetic testing really any different from blood or urine tests that are often ordered as a routine part of diagnosis? In this case, what constitutes informed consent?

What about when a healthy individual presents with a risk for some future disease and genetic testing is being used predictively? What constitutes informed consent in this case? Should a certain level of education about the disease and the test in question be required? And what is that level of education? How is this assessed? Does it make a difference if the disease is untreatable?

Should parents have the right to decide whether or not their child will have a genetic test? When a genetic test is used for diagnosis of symptoms, the issues are fairly straightforward because the child is already sick and the test is used to confirm the doctor's suspicions. The issues are also simpler when the test is being used to detect fairly common, very debilitating, highly treatable conditions such as PKU. In these cases, is consent measured differently?

Remember that neonatal screening procedures have been used nation-wide for years to detect and prevent a variety of common illnesses such as PKU or galactosemia. Would a genetic test for these or other similar diseases really be any different from the biochemical tests?

What about when a test is predictive of a future illness such as Huntington disease that is not apparent until later in life and is untreatable?

What if the person requesting genetic testing is very young? At what age can young people be expected to give informed consent for themselves—16, 18, 21? What standards should be applied in determining whether a child is qualified to make such a decision—age, emotional maturity, psychological maturity?

Many people believe that no individual should be tested presymptomatically or asymptomatically for genetic disease without first providing informed consent for the procedure. Many people also agree that young children are not able to fully provide informed consent, but this issue can become complicated.

Another aspect of informed consent involves genetic research. Frequently, DNA research and testing laboratories retain samples sent for testing for a period of time. This permits further testing of samples, if necessary, for comparison with additional family members who may present for testing at a later date. However, such samples can also be a valuable research tool. They provide a resource for large numbers of DNA samples from unrelated individuals. Having such a resource facilitates genetic research because it means that every time a scientist wants to test a population of samples they do not have to go out and collect them—the needed resources are already in the refrigerator in the lab. But under what circumstances can these samples be used for research purposes? If banking of

DNA is to be permitted, and if banked DNA samples are to be used in research, what precisely constitutes informed consent for this particular use of the samples?

Generally, scientists will remove all identifying labels from such samples before using them in research so that there is no way to trace the sample back to a particular person. But is the removal of all identifying labels prior to use of these samples sufficient to protect the patient? It is generally agreed that, if identifying labels are removed from samples, then use of banked DNA in research is acceptable and patients are adequately protected. DNA testing labs often include statements of consent on forms signed by patients so that the use of samples for research is permitted.

Finally, there is the question of genetic testing in conjunction with in vitro fertilization procedures. Take, for example, a couple with difficulty conceiving a child or a couple at high risk for having a child with a genetic disease. Suppose this couple requests in vitro fertilization to conceive a healthy child. There are available technologies that can test for genetic disease before implantation of fertilized embryos so that only healthy embryos, free of the genetic disease in question, will be implanted. This type of testing is called preimplantation diagnosis. The procedure has already seen limited application in the United States. If the parents are at risk for having a child with a given genetic disease, preimplantation testing can help reduce the risk that a child will be born carrying a debilitating disease. But should this couple also have the right to test for the sex of the child? What about other traits unrelated to disease?

Such complex and varied questions make education, medical genetic evaluation, and genetic counseling an important part of genetic testing for many people. Doctors and genetic counselors can often help patients in their search for information and options. Educating yourself about genetics and the benefits, implications, and limitations of genetic testing is important if you are to participate in and make informed choices about your own medical care.

Obviously, many of these issues are controversial, emotionally distressful, and complex. As such, there are no clear answers. People on opposite sides of the questions present compelling arguments in favor of their positions.

No doubt some answers will be objectionable to different groups for a variety of religious, social, or moral reasons, but they are questions that we as a society will be compelled to answer in the near future.

To this end, the Human Genome Project (discussed in some detail in Chapter 21) has developed a special committee called ELSI to study the ethical, legal, and social implications of genetic research. Today, more than eight million dollars per year of Human Genome Project money is spent to study these issues.

CHAPTER FIFTEEN

The Laboratory Practice
of Medical Genetics

Each genetic disease carries its own characteristic genetic alterations, biochemical characteristics, and diagnostic markers. Some genetic diseases can be diagnosed in the clinic based on the symptoms observed, with little or no need for genetic testing. For other genetic diseases the underlying genetic defect is still unknown, making traditional medical evaluation of patients the only diagnostic option.

However, there are many genetic diseases that can now be assessed at the level of DNA or protein in the genetics laboratory. And the number of diseases for which such precise laboratory tests are available is growing rapidly.

In addition to the clinician or genetic counselor that most patients see when consulting about concerns for a genetic disease, there are many different types of professionals who also work in the field of genetics. Many of these individuals work in the laboratory to develop and conduct the tests used to detect and diagnose genetic disease.

Three major fields of diagnostic genetics have developed out of the new technologies and the improved understanding of human genetics. These include cytogenetics, molecular genetics, and biochemical genetics.

Cytogenetics laboratories study genetic diseases caused by large alterations in the genome. Such diseases are detected as changes in the number or arrangement of chromosomes. Cytogeneticists use special methods to detect chromosomal alterations and aneuploidies.

Molecular genetics laboratories study genetic diseases caused by mutations in individual genes. Molecular geneticists use a variety of methods to detect the genetic alterations that affect individual genes.

Biochemical genetics laboratories study alterations in the biochemical or metabolic capabilities of cells that are caused by genetic disease. Biochemical geneticists use specialized methods to identify the metabolic disturbances within cells that are characteristic of genetic diseases.

The laboratory practice of genetics is a vital component of clinical genetics because it provides clinicians with additional resources for the complete evaluation of patients. In cases of complex or multifactorial diseases that can be caused by various types of alterations in the genome, genetic and biochemical diagnostic methods may soon become important in determining the precise cause of disease in a particular patient.

Each of these specialties and the tools they use to diagnose genetic disease are described in more detail in the next three chapters.

CHAPTER SIXTEEN

Cytogenetics

Cytogenetics ("cyto" meaning cell) is the field of study that examines the chromosomal makeup of cells. Cytogenetic diagnosis is performed on whole chromosomes. The aim is to examine the chromosomal content of cells. The goal is to detect aberrations in the chromosomal content of cells. Detection of certain chromosomal abnormalities can be diagnostic of particular genetic diseases.

The "karyotype" (pronounced CArry-o-type) is the primary method cytogeneticists use to examine the chromosomal content of cells. A karyotype is a method by which chromosomes are captured just before cell division and immobilized on glass slides for microscopic analysis.

Chromosomes for karyotype testing can be extracted from a variety of cell types and tissues including amniotic fluid, chorionic villus sampling, or blood. When amniocentesis is performed during pregnancy for chromosomal analysis of a fetus to screen for Down syndrome or to determine the sex of the child, a karyotype is the typical way that such an analysis is conducted.

During karyotype preparation, the chromosomes are stained with a dye that generates a characteristic alternating pattern of light and dark stripes, or bands, on each different chromosome. Following staining, chromosomes are labeled by chromosome number and by band. First, chromosomes are designated with a particular chromosome number based on their length and staining pattern. Next, the chromosomes are divided into segments and the individual bands are labeled.

The band segments are located using an easily identifiable chromosomal feature called the "centromere." The centromere is the part of the chromosome involved in cell division that helps the chromosomes assort to each of the newly forming cells. The centromere appears on a karyotype as a narrowed region along the rod length of the chromosome. On each side of the centromere is an arm of the chromosome. The shorter of the two arms is called the "p" arm, and the longer arm is called the "q" arm.

The pattern of bands produced by the dye stain on the chromosome arms is used as a guide to label the bands numerically. Band numbers increase as the bands move out from the centromere toward the ends of the chromosomes. This precise labeling is necessary so that doctors and scientists can detect abnormalities and communicate specific alterations in a universal, common language.

Analysis of the banding pattern for each patient's sample can allow the detection of chromosomal abnormalities. Karyotyping can be used to detect

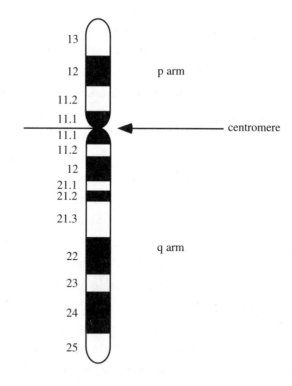

FIGURE 16.1   Diagram of chromosome 17 with the centromere, p and q arms, and individual cytogenetic bands labeled. Bands are labeled for each arm individually, starting at the centromere and working outward. Note that the band numbers do not necessarily follow a consecutive numbering system.

many types of chromosomal alterations such as deletion mutations, insertion or duplication mutations, inversions, and translocations. These alterations are detected by observing a disruption in normal chromosome banding patterns. Karyotype analysis can also be used to detect chromosomal aneuploidies such as Down syndrome and Turner syndrome. These are detected through observation of extra or missing chromosomal material.

Many genetic diseases are characterized by specific chromosomal defects. Discovery of three chromosome 21s in a sample indicates Down syndrome, while Prader-Willi and Angelman syndromes can often be diagnosed by the loss of bands 11 to 13 from the q (long) arm of chromosome 15.

Today, more advanced methods for cytogenetic analysis are frequently used in laboratories. These methods, which include chromosome painting and fluorescent in situ hybridization (FISH), represent an improvement in technology. They can detect small alterations that might not be detected with the more conventional karyotyping technologies. They can also be used to assess precisely the nature of a complex or uncharacteristic chromosome alteration.

The new methods use DNA probes to pinpoint a particular segment of the genome. DNA probes are small pieces of DNA that are designed and made in the laboratory. DNA probes take advantage of the base pairing that occurs between the two sides of a DNA ladder.

DNA probes are like magnets. They are identical in DNA sequence to the region of DNA that a scientist wants to study and are tagged with fluorescent or radioactive material that makes them easy to detect. The DNA probes are then used to specifically seek out, bind to, and enhance certain parts of the genome.

In chromosome painting and FISH, DNA probes give scientists a better view of specific chromosomal regions. Using DNA probes, very small alterations in the chromosomes can be detected. Additional applications of DNA probes are discussed in detail in Chapter 19.

Finally, cytogenetic analysis can be used to study characteristic genetic changes found in certain types of cancer such as leukemia. The specific genetic changes found in cancer cells can sometimes tell doctors a great deal about the type of cancer present, the prognosis for the patient, and possible treatment approaches.

CHAPTER SEVENTEEN

Molecular Genetics

For the molecular diagnosis of genetic disease, tests are performed on individual genes instead of on whole chromosomes. The aim of molecular diagnostics is to determine the DNA sequence of genes. The goal is to detect changes in the DNA sequence that cause genetic disease.

Molecular genetic testing uses purified DNA that has been extracted from cells. To extract DNA, cells are popped open in a water-based solution, releasing the DNA. After a series of purification steps in which the DNA is separated from the remaining cellular material such as the proteins, the extracted DNA is used in molecular tests.

Some types of molecular tests require extensive purification of large amounts of DNA. Other types of tests may work well on crude, less pure extracts. DNA can be extracted from a variety of cell types and tissues including cells from amniotic fluid, chorionic villus sampling, biopsy samples, blood, dried blood spots, or buccal cell (cheek) swabs. The testing procedure to be performed and the amount of DNA required often dictates the type and size of samples to be taken from a patient.

Diseases for which molecular analysis is most useful are those in which the responsible gene has been identified and sequenced, and in which mutations can be readily detected. Presently, molecular genetic analysis is available for many genetic diseases, and most tests are highly reliable. Cystic fibrosis, Tay-Sachs disease, Gaucher disease, Duchenne muscular dystrophy, sickle cell disease, fragile X mental retardation, Huntington disease, hemophilia, and myotonic dystrophy are just a few examples of genetic diseases that can be diagnosed using molecular methods. As the ability to detect DNA mutations rapidly improves and as new genes are discovered, many more genetic diseases will be amenable to diagnosis using molecular genetic methods.

A number of laboratory techniques can be used to find mutations that result in genetic disease. Different laboratory methods are used to detect deletions, insertions, inversions, point mutations, or other rearrangements. The methods chosen will depend upon the suspected diagnosis and the mutations characteristic to that particular disease. As a result, molecular genetic laboratories will often employ a variety of different testing methods.

Molecular genetic methods use DNA probes to seek out and enhance certain genetic elements and separate the gene of interest from the rest of the DNA in a sample. DNA probes in molecular genetics are small pieces of DNA that have been made in the lab and carry the same sequence as the gene of interest. The probes are labeled with a fluorescent or radioactive substance to make them easy to detect and are then introduced into the DNA sample taken from the patient and allowed to base pair with the DNA in the sample. With its fluorescent or radioactive tag, the probe's binding to the sample enhances the ability to see the sequence of the DNA being tested.

Molecular genetic methods can also be used for other purposes such as forensic analysis, personal identification, and paternity testing. As we have already learned, no two people—with the exception of identical twins—share exactly the same DNA.

For forensic analysis, personal identification, or paternity testing, the basic goal is the same. Molecular genetic testing methods are used to compare DNA sequences between different people. The aim is to detect the individual variations in DNA sequence that normally occur between people. Remember, not all genetic variations among people are indicative of genetic disease.

Normal variations in DNA sequence occur throughout the genome, but are especially common in the parts of the genome that do not make genes. Changes in these regions of DNA, since they do not code for proteins, are not likely to be functionally important to cells. Therefore, the DNA sequence is not as tightly controlled in these regions as it is in others because there is no apparent adverse effect of changes in the sequence.

On the other hand, the regions of the DNA that encode genes generally do not vary much from person to person. That is because variation might result in the manufacture of a protein that does not work properly, impairing the survival of the individual. As a result, the likelihood that any two people would share a DNA sequence within the protein encoding portion of a gene is high, and these less variable regions of the DNA are not as useful for distinguishing among individuals. Since the goal of personal identification, forensic DNA testing, and paternity testing is to detect differences in the DNA, it is best to study regions of the DNA that vary from person to person. Scientists have conducted extensive research to identify the best regions of the genome to use for these purposes.

Having identified specific regions of the DNA that commonly vary from person to person, researchers then compare samples taken from large numbers of people and from people of different ethnic backgrounds. This research allows scientists to identify all the possible DNA sequences that can be found at any given site in the genome. By characterizing the DNA sequence differences in large numbers of people, scientists can determine the frequency with which any one variation or allele occurs. The frequency of each allele is also measured for different ethnic groups to assess whether there are differences in the frequency of alleles in different populations. This research is necessary so that the calculations used to estimate probabilities are as accurate as possible.

The population frequencies of each allele are used to determine the likelihood that any two people will share a DNA sequence at a particular site. Take for example, an imaginary sequence on chromosome 1. Say there are two variations on that sequence that are found among all the people tested. Let's call these alleles sequence A and sequence B.

For the purposes of this example, let's suppose that each of these alleles, A and B, occur with equal frequency in the population of individuals tested. That is, allele A occurs 50 percent of the time in the population and allele B occurs 50 percent of the time in the population. So, if you studied one hundred people at random, each with two copies of chromosome 1 in their cells, you would be studying two hundred total chromosome 1s, and you would find sequence B one hundred times and sequence A one hundred times.

Since each person carries two chromosome 1s, each will carry two copies of the sequence. As a result, some people will carry only sequence A—that is, sequence A on both of their chromosome 1s. Their genotype would be AA. Some people will carry only sequence B—that is, sequence B on both of their chromosome 1s. Their genotype would be BB. And some people will carry both sequences A and B—that is, sequence A on one of their chromosome 1s and sequence B on the other. Their genotype would be either AB or BA.

Since we know that both alleles occur with equal frequency (50 percent or 0.5), we can calculate the likelihood of each genotype, AA, AB, BA, and BB. Since AB and BA will look identical on a DNA test, they are grouped together.

With these numbers, we can calculate that 25 percent of people will be genotype AA (0.5 A times 0.5 A). Twenty-five percent of people will be BB (0.5 B times 0.5 B) and 50 percent of people will be AB (25 percent AB plus 25 percent BA).

Now let's use this sequence to see if the DNA from a suspect matches the DNA from a crime scene. If we collect DNA from a crime scene and it tests to be AA, then we are looking for a suspect who does not carry a B allele. That is, a suspect who is neither BB nor AB. If a suspect carries a B allele, that suspect can be ruled out.

Since the AA genotype occurs in 25 percent of the population, 25 percent of the population would be included by the test as possible suspects. If only this one site were used to distinguish between several different people, it would only work 75 percent of the time. Twenty five percent of the time, two people would have the same sequence and would be indistinguishable genetically simply by chance and not by guilt. Those are not very powerful odds.

However, if many different sites in the genome are compared instead of just one, then the likelihood that any two people would continue to share the exact same DNA sequence at every site tested decreases dramatically with each successive site tested. This is because somewhere along the line, a difference in sequence is likely to be found, unless the two people are identical twins.

Take for example a case where two independent sites are tested, each with the same profile as the site described above. The ability to distinguish between people would be 25 percent (1 in 4) for the first site times 25 percent (1 in 4) for the second site. Now the ability of the test to distinguish among people goes to 1 in 4 times 1 in 4 or 1 in 16 (1 in 4^2). This result yields a 1 in 16 chance that two people, by chance, would share exactly the same genotype at both sites.

Add a third independent site to the test, and it becomes 1 in 4 times 1 in 4 times 1 in 4 or 1 in 64 (1 in 4^3). With each site tested, the ability of the test to distinguish among individuals increases. Test ten independent sites with the same characteristics as the example above, and the odds of two people sharing the same DNA sequences at every site becomes 1 in 4^{10}—or better than one in one million.

By testing enough separate sites in the genome, the likelihood that any two people would share the same DNA sequences at every site tested can become remarkably low. The more sites that are tested and matched between a sample of DNA at a crime scene and a suspect, for example, the more likely it is that the DNA sample taken from the crime scene came from that suspect.

When the odds are given in a court case that the DNA in a sample came from a particular suspect, the numbers are a cumulative statistical probability—based on the data gathered about the DNA sites tested—that any two people, chosen at random, would share the same DNA sequence at every one of the many sites.

However, readers should keep in mind a few things. First, this example used sites with similar genotype frequencies. Few, if any, DNA polymorphisms used in forensic applications will be exactly alike. Usually, the sites chosen for forensic DNA testing have several alleles. The additional alleles can dramatically increase the power of sites to distinguish among individuals. And since this is a very simplified example, provided for illustrative purposes only, it is important to point out that the calculations in real cases are quite a bit more complex.

But what if differences in the DNA sequence between the sample and the suspect are found? Then the possibility that the two DNA samples came from the same person is ruled out. In this way, DNA can be used like dental records or fingerprints as a form of identification for individuals.

The types of molecular genetic methods that are used to detect differences in DNA between people are sometimes referred to as DNA fingerprinting. Just like the types of fingerprinting that we normally think of with an ink blot and paper where ridges in the tips of the fingers are used to distinguish between individuals, the genetic methods use differences in DNA sequence to distinguish among individuals.

For forensic DNA analysis, DNA can be extracted from bodily fluids or tissue samples such as blood, semen, skin, or hair found at or associated with crime scenes. The samples are DNA fingerprinted and compared to the DNA fingerprint of suspects and victims. The more genetic locations at which the DNA sequences are compared and found to be identical with those of a suspect, the greater the likelihood that the two samples came from the same person. If the samples are pivotal evidence in the crime scene, then the more likely it is that the suspect was present at the scene. However, if DNA sequence differences are found between a sample of evidence and a suspect, it suggests that the sample did not come from the suspect.

Forensic DNA technology can be used in animals, as well. For example, in 1993 there was a report by Guglich, Wilson, and White in the Journal of Forensic Sciences that DNA fingerprinting technology had been used in Ontario, Canada, by the forest and wildlife service to identify a suspect in illegal hunting activities. In this case, DNA was extracted from blood spots collected at a site where hunting was illegal. This DNA was compared to DNA extracted from meat found in the suspect's freezer. Comparison of the samples revealed that the two DNA samples had come from the same animal. This provided the basis for positive identification of the individual who had been suspected in illegal hunting.

Forensic DNA technology can also be used to detect bacterial and viral DNA patterns among samples such as food and soil.

For personal identification, DNA can be extracted from individuals, characterized, and either compared with relatives or stored in a database or archive for later retrieval. Then, if a circumstance arises where the source of bodily remains or blood spots needs to be identified, the DNA fingerprint data from the sample can be compared to the family samples or the computer database to confirm the identity of the individual from which the sample came. Possible applications of this technology include: identification of unknown human remains in time of war, missing persons, or criminal investigations; profiling of precise histologic genetic information for identifying potential organ donors from a database; and databasing of DNA profiles from convicted criminals for retrieval in future investigations of crime scenes.

There are two recent, widely publicized examples of DNA tests being used to identify persons. In one case, DNA testing helped to confirm the identity of the soldier buried in the Tomb of the Unknowns in Washington, D.C. In another case, DNA tests confirmed the identity of the remains of Czar Nicholas and his family in a grave in Russia.

For paternity testing, the goal of DNA analysis is to determine whether an alleged father made a genetic contribution to a child. In these cases, DNA is extracted from the mother, the child, and the alleged father, either from a blood sample or a cheek swab. The DNA from the mother is compared with that from the child to identify which of the child's DNA sequences at each test site were inherited from the mother. The remaining sites are then compared to the alleged father's DNA pattern. If it is found that the child carries identical sequences at the test sites to those carried by the alleged father, then paternity becomes increasingly likely with each additional site tested. If, however, the child carries DNA sequences that could not have come from the alleged father, then doubt is cast on the genetic contribution of that man to the child and paternity can be ruled out. The use of DNA fingerprinting technologies for paternity testing has become widespread because of its high accuracy, sensitivity, and specificity.

The application of molecular genetic methods to personal identification, forensics, and paternity testing is expected to continue to increase.

CHAPTER EIGHTEEN

Biochemical Genetics

Biochemical genetic analysis does not study genes or chromosomes directly, but instead asks questions about the biochemical or enzymatic makeup of cells. The aim is to examine the metabolic capacity of cells. The goal is to identify aberrations in the metabolic process. The presence or absence of certain enzymes, proteins, or chemical compounds can be diagnostic of certain genetic diseases.

As we have already learned, enzymes are proteins that perform metabolic reactions in cells and catalyze the biochemical conversion of one chemical substance to another. Many genetic diseases are due to defects in enzymes. These defective enzymes cause a malfunction in the metabolic capabilities of cells. When an enzyme does not work because of a genetic defect, many things can happen. For example, cells may lack an important substance that is the product of the enzymatic process. On the other hand, the lack of an enzyme can result in the buildup of a participant in the enzymatic process that is not normally present in large amounts.

FIGURE 18.1 Diagram showing the results of an enzymatic defect. In the diagram on the left, in the presence of the enzyme, compound A is readily converted to compound B. On the right, in the absence of the enzyme, compound A builds up and compound B is missing.

147

In some cases, enzyme activities are measured directly, and in other cases, metabolic products are identified and measured. For example, the deficiency of Hexosaminidase A (Hex A), which causes Tay-Sachs disease, is often measured by assessment of the actual level of enzyme activity in a sample. Alternatively, the deficiency of the enzyme phenylalanine hydrox-ylase, which causes PKU, is measured by assessment of the level of phenyl-lalanine in blood. Phenylalanine is a component of the reaction that builds up in the blood when there is a lack of enzyme activity.

Biochemical genetics laboratories use precise instruments to detect chem-ical components of cells and to measure enzyme activities. Biochemical analysis can be performed on a variety of tissues or samples, including blood, urine, cerebrospinal fluid (CSF), amniotic fluid, CVS samples, and dried blood spots. The patient samples required and the methods chosen generally reflect the suspected diagnosis. Biochemical testing provides a rapid, reliable screen for the diagnostic confirmation of many diseases.

Sometimes biochemical testing can be used to assist other methods such as molecular diagnostics. For example, molecular testing can only detect the mutations for which it scans, but biochemical testing can address the overall function of an enzyme, regardless of what particular mutation it car-ries. In this case, biochemical analysis facilitates diagnosis.

On the other hand, in the case of carrier screening for enzyme defects, biochemical analysis may sometimes be assisted by another method such as DNA testing. One reason for this is because carriers of mutations in one allele of a gene pair will still have one normal gene and will produce some amount of functioning enzyme. Reduced amounts of enzyme may be diffi-cult in some cases to distinguish from normal levels by biochemical meth-ods, and another testing approach may be helpful in the identification of unaffected carriers. In other cases, the biochemical test may not always yield conclusive results because some naturally occurring enzyme variants may not test well in the laboratory. These variants, while not associated with disease, may appear equivocal upon laboratory testing, giving a false pos-itive result. Consequently, a combination of techniques including biochemical and molecular genetic methods may be used for the complete characterization of a family.

The X-linked recessive disease Lesch-Nyhan syndrome is an example of a genetic condition in which a combination of techniques is sometimes used for diagnosis. The syndrome is caused by a deficiency of the enzyme hypoxanthine guanine phosphoribosyl-transferase (HGPRT or HPRT) and is characterized by gout, mental retardation, choreoathetosis (a type of fluctuating muscle tone resulting in involuntary movements), and self-mutilatory behavior. The deficiency of HPRT in affected males is most easily measured using biochemical methods. However, carrier testing for identification of carrier females using biochemical methods is not always straightforward, and molecular genetic methods can sometimes provide a more definitive assessment of carrier status.

CHAPTER NINETEEN

How Genetic Research and Testing Is Done

In genetic research, as in any other type of scientific inquiry, scientists are dependent on their tools to be able to ask and answer questions. At its most basic level, genetic research is about studying genes. In order to find and study a gene, researchers must be able to separate gene-containing segments of DNA so small that they cannot be seen from all the other DNA of a cell, which also cannot be seen. Finding a single gene in the context of the entire human genome is very much like looking for a needle in a haystack. It would help if you had a magnet!

Scientists have a variety of different laboratory tools that they utilize to study DNA. All are based on a few simple principles that take advantage of the basic structure of DNA—principles that we have already discussed in this book. For example, we have learned that DNA likes to be double stranded, and that the sequence of one side of the DNA strand predicts the sequence of the other. We have also learned that DNA is copied within the cell, and that there are proteins inside cells made specifically for that purpose—proteins that can be isolated and used in the laboratory. Finally, scientists have discovered enzymes, made by bacteria, that can cut the DNA ladder reliably at very specific sequences. These four basic principles of DNA give scientists the tools they need to make DNA in the laboratory, separate small pieces of DNA from the whole genomic content, and use one piece of DNA as bait to find another.

In genetic research, the four basic principles of DNA described here can be used to do many things, including identify, isolate, clone, and sequence genes. Much of the current effort in genetic research is geared toward cloning genes. Unlike the cloning of Dolly, the Scottish sheep whose birth was so widely reported in the news, the cloning of individual genes does not involve the production of whole animals. Instead, when genes are cloned they are separated from the rest of the genomic material of a cell and introduced into a genetic background in which they can be studied more easily, like a bacteria or a virus.

When cloning a gene or part of a chromosome, typically the first step is to purify the whole amount of DNA in a cell away from the rest of the components of the cell such as the proteins. The purified DNA is then cut up or digested by one of the special bacterial enzymes that can break DNA at specific sequences. Digestion of the DNA of a cell with these bacterial enzymes results in hundreds of thousands—and in some cases millions—of small fragments of DNA. These fragments of DNA are then introduced separately into the genetic material of a bacterium, yeast cell, or virus.

When completed, this process results in the creation of what is called a genomic library. Literally, it is a batch of bacteria, viruses, or yeast that among their population carry a large portion of the human genetic material in tiny, separate pieces. The entire collection represents the genetic library of a human cell. Similar libraries of genetic sequences called cDNA libraries are made from the total RNA content of a cell rather than the DNA content. Genomic and cDNA libraries can be made from any type of cell or tissue from any organism.

A genomic library contains most of the DNA of a cell. A cDNA library, which is made from the RNA of a cell, is enriched for expressed genes only. The cDNA libraries are used in research to identify and characterize expressed genes and to compare gene expression between different types of cells or tissues. For example, comparing the contents of a cDNA library made from a liver cell with the contents of a cDNA library made from a muscle cell can help a scientist detect differences in gene expression between the two cell types. If a genetic disease affects liver cells but not muscle cells, finding proteins that are used in liver and not in muscle might provide a good place to start looking for the genetic defect. Alternatively, if a gene is found in a liver cell that is suspected of causing liver disease, examining its expression in other tissues can sometimes help explain the profile of symptoms seen in the disease and identify other organs at risk.

Once isolated and introduced into these simpler biological systems, human genes can be grown rapidly because bacteria, viruses, and yeast replicate very quickly. The individual genes that have been introduced into a bacterium or virus or yeast are said to be cloned. The cloned DNA can be easily purified because bacteria, viruses, and yeast have far less DNA than human cells. This relative purification makes studying a gene easier and provides scientists with more effective ways to ask questions about a gene's function or what happens to a cell if a gene is mutated.

Clearly, the cloning of genes does not require the reproduction of whole animals. This type of cloning is crucial to the study and understanding of human genes and genetic diseases. Without the ability to clone genes, we would not have the understanding of genetics, biology, or medicine that we do today, nor would the science progress at its current rate. We would also not be likely to achieve the advances in medicine that are sure to come from genetic research.

The cloning of a gene into a bacterium, virus, or yeast also provides another advantage: It allows for a relatively pure source of the protein that the gene encodes. Bacteria and yeast can be forced to produce huge quantities of RNA and protein from the cloned gene, and this material can be easily isolated, purified, and studied.

Such cloned, purified proteins are the basis for production of many of the therapeutic proteins that we have today. For example, human growth hormone and Factor VIII need no longer be purified from human tissue but instead can be mass produced in cloned systems. Human growth hormone is sometimes used to treat certain forms of dwarfism and other human conditions where short stature is a symptom. Factor VIII is used to treat Hemophilia A. Cloning of the gene and protein makes for a much purer, safer source of the protein for therapeutic applications because of the reduced risk of contamination from human infectious agents.

In research and testing for genetic disease, the fact that the DNA ladder has two sides has several advantages. It allows scientists to know the sequence of both sides of the ladder after determining the sequence of only one side. In addition, the double-stranded ladder is very easy to break apart. All you have to do is warm up the DNA or put it in a highly alkaline (high pH) solution. When this is done, the DNA ladder literally splits apart into its two independent sides and becomes single stranded. These two features of DNA allow scientists to develop and use DNA probes. As discussed in Chapters 16 and 17, DNA probes are pieces of DNA that are identical to a particular sequence of DNA that is of interest, such as a gene. Scientists can use these probes to pinpoint the location of a specific gene in a population of DNA.

In the lab, DNA ladders in a sample are forced apart with heat or high pH, creating single-stranded DNA and the opportunity for new base pairing or new ladders to form. Another piece of DNA, one that is made in the lab and is labeled with some kind of substance that makes it visible (a fluorescent dye or radioactivity), can be used like a magnet to seek out its complement among the rest of the DNA pieces in the sample. The DNA probe will bind to its complement in the single-stranded sample and light it up, giving scientists the ability to distinguish that segment of DNA from all the other DNA in the sample.

Sometimes this approach is used in the context of whole chromosomes, as described in Chapter 16. For example, if you want to study the region of chromosome 15 that is frequently deleted, or lost, in Prader-Willi and Angelman syndromes, you could take a piece of DNA in the lab that has the same sequence as the DNA ladder in this region of chromosome 15 and label it with a fluorescent dye. Then you could combine the labeled DNA with cytogenetic karyotype analysis. You would make a slide of chromosomes from a patient's sample and mix your fluorescent DNA with it, forcing the two DNAs to bind together.

Since there are two chromosome 15s per cell, the karyotype microscope slide should have two fluorescent dots on it—one for each chromosome 15 in a cell. If only one fluorescent dot is found per cell, that means a deletion of that region from one of the chromosome 15s has occurred, suggesting genetic disease. Whether it is Prader-Willi or Angelman syndrome will depend upon whether the chromosome inherited from the mother or the chromosome inherited from the father carries the deletion, as was described in Chapter 11.

The same basic approach is used to study precise mutations in individual genes. DNA probes are used to visualize the DNA of one gene apart from the DNA in the rest of the genome. The DNA probes are either radioactively or fluorescently labeled and mixed with the sample DNA to determine if a gene's sequence characteristics coincide with a normal sequence or a disease-related sequence.

In one type of procedure called "allele-specific oligonucleotide (ASO) hybridization," the normal sequence and the mutated sequence are both used as probes. The ability of both sequences to bind to the DNA in the sample is compared. If the mutant sequence binds and the normal sequence does not, then it is assumed that the person does not carry a normal sequence in that gene. If the disease in question is recessive, the person would be predicted to be affected. In recessive diseases, if the normal sequence binds and the mutant sequence does not, the person is not likely to be affected and also is not likely to be a carrier of the disease. However, if both normal and mutant sequences bind, then the person is likely to carry both a normal and a mutant gene and is presumed to be a carrier. On the other hand, if the disease is dominant and both normal and mutant probes bind to the DNA in the sample, then the patient would be presumed to be affected.

Scientists can make mutant gene probes if the DNA sequences of genes and the common disease-causing mutations are known. The accuracy of a DNA test will depend on the number of disease alleles involved and the likelihood of finding a mutation in a certain human population. For example, ASO analysis is frequently used to diagnose patients and detect unaffected carriers for cystic fibrosis (CF). A number of common CF mutations have been characterized and can be detected by ASO analysis using a separate DNA probe for each mutation. The percentage of CF patients that carry these known mutations for a variety of human populations has been experimentally determined. Knowing the likelihood of detecting a disease gene in a given population permits calculation of genetic risk.

For ASO CF testing, the DNA sample taken from a person is subjected to analysis with both normal and mutant sequence DNA probes. If both sequences bind to the DNA sample from the person, and if that person is healthy, then he or she is presumed with reasonable likelihood to be an unaffected carrier. If only the mutant sequences bind to the DNA sample from the person, and if the person is showing symptoms of CF, then he or she is presumed to be affected by CF. If only the normal sequences bind to the DNA from the person, then that person is presumed to have a low risk of being a carrier. The risk is never zero, however, because some rare mutation that the test cannot detect might still be present.

Remember, you can only find mutations that you test for. Other mutations are not usually detected serendipitously by a test such as this. However, the likelihood of someone being a carrier can be revealed by these types of tests, especially if the individual has a family history of the disease and the mutation in the affected individuals can be identified. If you know the mutations that caused the disease in the affected family member, then you can look specifically for that mutation in close relatives. If that mutation is absent in the relatives tested for carrier status, then their carrier risk may be lowered. Depending upon the number of mutations the test is designed to detect and the family history and ethnic background of the patient, exact risk estimates will vary. As such, it is important that patients ask for a clear description of their carrier risk and disease risk, and a precise calculation of the likelihood of each.

In another type of DNA analysis, called a "Southern analysis," the DNA is cut up into smaller pieces—or digested—using bacterial enzymes. The pieces are then separated by size, and a DNA probe is used to find the gene of interest. Southern analysis is useful for genes in which changes in length of the DNA sequence are indicative of disease as well as for genes in which the disease-causing mutation interrupts enzyme's the ability to cut DNA. Southern analysis can also detect rearrangements in the structure of a gene that cause changes in the size of a portion of the gene. In each of these circumstances, the DNA in the test sample will be a different size than would be expected because of the mutation.

In both genetic research and testing, scientists often need to enrich the amount of a particular DNA sequence in a sample. The "polymerase chain reaction," or PCR, is a relatively new technology that has revolutionized the study of DNA in the laboratory. This approach uses enzymes for replicating DNA (much like a copier machine) to amplify a particular sequence of DNA millions of times in just a few hours. Enriching a DNA sample for a particular gene sequence provides scientists with a larger supply of material to study and vastly improves the ability to detect and analyze mutations. PCR is used frequently in DNA laboratories today. PCR is especially useful in forensic DNA analysis in which the amount of DNA in a sample may be very low. For example, if evidence such as blood spots are collected from a crime scene, the spots may be small and therefore may not contain much DNA. PCR is used to amplify the DNA so that there is enough material for DNA testing.

Sometimes the entire DNA sequence of a gene has to be studied in order to identify disease-causing mutations. Usually, the genes that require this approach are the ones in which there are few if any commonly occurring mutations. In these cases, every patient generally carries his or her own unique mutation. Such personally unique mutations make generalized mutation detection difficult because no two patients are likely to carry exactly the same mutation, and because standardized tests do not have a high rate of return. To sequence genes, scientists use DNA-replicating enzymes to synthesize new fragments of DNA from the gene of interest and study the resulting DNA sequence. The DNA sequence from the patient is compared to the normal gene sequence in an effort to detect disease-causing mutations. This type of DNA testing is called DNA sequencing and is often time consuming, labor intensive, and expensive to perform. New technologies currently under development may make the detection of unique disease mutations more efficient, reducing the time and cost of this type of DNA test.

The field of genetic research and testing is a complicated endeavor. Scientists spend a lot of time in the laboratory mastering the tools of their trade. This chapter described only a few of the methods available to today's sophisticated research and testing laboratories.

In any type of genetic analysis, as in other medical testing, extenuating circumstances can occasionally alter the reliability or predictive value of the test results. Genetic testing of any kind should always be conducted by qualified laboratories, and test results should always be evaluated by qualified, highly trained professionals to reduce the chance of inappropriate testing and misinterpretation of test results.

CHAPTER TWENTY

The Importance of Genetic Research

The federal government and private research foundations combine to spend hundreds of millions of dollars every year on genetic research. With this kind of price tag, the expectation for meaningful contribution to people's lives is tremendous. So what does genetic research really do for us?

Advances in Biology and Medicine

The most basic contribution of genetic research is that it teaches us about how our bodies work, how they grow and develop, and what happens when something goes wrong from the inside. Just like a mechanic working on a car, a doctor needs to know how the body works when it works right to be able to fix it when something goes wrong. The basic knowledge gained from genetic research is necessary if we are to continue to develop and enrich medical knowledge.

For example, consider congenital heart defects. Congenital heart defects occur in about 0.8 percent of births in the United States. Many of these defects have a genetic or multifactorial cause. While surgery is often used to try to repair congenital heart defects, we still do not know on a cellular level why many of these defects occur. In other words, we do not have a good understanding of why the cells in one heart did not grow together the way cells in another heart did. And we do not know on the most basic level how a defect in a particular gene can cause a defect in a heart, or whatever other organ may be disrupted by a gene defect.

159

For congenital heart defects, we can try to repair the mechanical workings of the heart, but there is little we can do to prevent recurrence of the
defect in another child. Learning about the way genes work to develop a
heart will provide insight into how the heart grows from conception to
adulthood and how alterations in genes or certain environmental factors
may interfere with that process. The hope is that this knowledge eventually
will lead to more effective medical interventions to repair defects and
maybe even prevent them. This approach to medical genetic research is currently being applied to countless human traits, conditions, and disorders.

Advances in Technology

Genetic research also provides us with advances in medical technology.
More and more frequently doctors are being provided with new molecular
or biochemical tools that they can use to diagnose and treat their patients.

For example, there are now several types of neurologic disease for which
the genetic basis has been identified. Many of these diseases can present
with overlapping symptoms. As such, precise diagnosis in early stages may
not always be straightforward. The new availability of precise genetic tests
for many of these diseases allows doctors to diagnose patients based on the
presence or absence of a specific genetic defect. This allows doctors to rule
out some syndromes and accurately diagnose others. Precise diagnosis is
always important for patient care, prediction of the course of a disease, and
estimation of risk that other family members may get the disease.

On another level, genetic research is providing advances in computer
software and information management. Computer programs are being
developed that will make it easier to store and distribute the massive
amounts of data now being deposited in databases around the world.
Programs are also being developed to help scientists analyze and interpret
data. The technology of information management is called informatics.
Advances in informatics are providing new computing capabilities that are
likely to have applications beyond genetics.

Gene Discovery

Historically, genetic research had gone on quietly in labs around the world, with very few people knowing much about the successes unless something occurred that was of widespread interest. Today, however, the successes of genetic research are often met with quite a bit of media publicity.

One of the most visible results of genetic research is the discovery of a gene—exciting events that come after years of painstaking research. Newspapers and television news networks often carry stories about newly found genes. Unfortunately, media coverage of the discovery of a gene is usually short lived, and people can become disillusioned when cures are not immediately forthcoming.

True, the discovery of a gene is always cause for optimism, but we must not forget that discovery of a gene will usually not lead to an instant treatment or cure. Take for example, the genes that cause cystic fibrosis (CF) and Duchenne muscular dystrophy (DMD). These genes were found several years ago, with a great flurry of enthusiasm. But still, years later, cures have yet to be achieved. For patients, families, and researchers alike, this is frustrating, and we must remember that even though the discovery of a gene does not lead to an immediate cure, it is a great step in that direction.

What gene discovery does is to provide scientists with the necessary materials to study how a gene works. Having a gene in hand gives scientists a tool for making the encoded protein in the laboratory. Having a protein in large quantities gives scientists a chance to study the protein's size, shape, and function. Understanding the function of a protein allows scientists to learn about the effect of changes in the protein and how mutations in the gene bring those changes about.

Having a protein also provides the raw material for locating the protein within a cell and determining its site of action. Learning where in a cell the protein works, what other proteins it works with, and how changes in the protein affect a cell gives scientists insight into the biological causes behind the symptoms of a genetic disease.

In addition to studying genes in model laboratory systems, genetic research is advanced by having patient materials to study. The participation of patient volunteers and their relatives is important because these individuals provide valuable samples for analysis. Patient samples can give scientists resources not only for discovering genes but also for comparing how affected tissues and unaffected tissues are different. This provides insight into the medical implications for a patient carrying a particular genetic mutation.

Ultimately, the hope of genetic research is that successes will lead doctors and scientists toward new and improved methods for treatment of genetic diseases. Today, it is common that the genes involved in genetic diseases are found long before we have any knowledge about what the proteins encoded by those genes do. As a result, the ability to diagnose a disease often precedes the ability to treat. But the future of molecular medicine will be not just in the ability to diagnose a genetic disease rapidly and accurately, but also to prevent or cure it.

Take for example the story of Duchenne muscular dystrophy or DMD. DMD is an X-linked recessive disorder that causes extreme muscle weakness and respiratory difficulty in affected patients. Being X-linked recessive, the disease usually affects males. Affected males are generally wheelchair bound by their teens and eventually succumb to respiratory failure.

For many years, the biochemical basis of the muscle deterioration seen with this disease was unknown. Cloning of the gene in 1987 led to the development of genetic tests for the detection of disease-causing mutations and provided a source for producing the DMD protein. Having the gene and protein in hand gave scientists the materials needed to study how mutations in the gene result in the muscular degeneration seen in patients.

Because of these early discoveries, scientists now know where in muscle cells the DMD protein is found, what role the protein plays in muscle cell structure and function, and why gene mutations cause muscle weakness and respiratory failure. The new, deeper understanding of this protein and of muscle tissue in general has led to the discovery of previously unknown proteins that are associated with the DMD protein. These discoveries have allowed the rapid characterization of other, related genetic disorders.

Now the challenge with DMD and related disorders is to try to develop more effective treatments. Since we have learned the who, what, where and why of DMD, we can begin to ask new questions. What if we could treat this disease? How would we do that effectively? Research into new treatment approaches such as gene therapy is already making significant early strides toward the development of effective treatments for DMD and many other genetic diseases.

CHAPTER TWENTY-ONE

The Human Genome Project

The Human Genome Project is a large-scale, international, biological science research effort designed to decipher the genetic information of man and many other organisms. In the United States, the Human Genome Project is led by the National Institutes of Health (NIH) and the Department of Energy (DOE). Other participants include the National Science Foundation (NSF), the Howard Hughes Medical Institute (HHMI), and the United States Department of Agriculture (USDA). The project has established genome research centers throughout the country for executing its goals. The international genome effort is coordinated by the Human Genome Organization (HUGO) and involves nearly 20 countries.

The level of funding in the United States for the project has increased every year since 1988. In 1998, the Human Genome Project received over $300 million in NIH and DOE funding. The intensive coordination of the project makes this approach cheaper, faster, and more efficient than a less organized approach. Coordination avoids redundant or competing projects and facilitates data and technology sharing among cooperating laboratories.

The project has numerous goals and far-reaching implications. It is predicted that the information gathered from the human genome project will revolutionize the practice of medicine in the next century. It will advance our understanding of the role genes play in human health and illness. It will provide new approaches to the diagnosis, treatment, and prevention of genetic diseases. It will provide technological advances that can be applied to a number of different fields. And it will raise social and ethical issues never before faced by mankind.

Among the scientific goals of the project are the construction of genetic and physical maps of the human genome. Genetic maps are diagrammatic representations of where specific DNA sequences called markers reside on chromosomes. Markers are like tags or street signs on chromosomes that provide points on the genetic road map. Markers represent specific traits, diseases, or unique DNA sequences. The goal of genetic mapping is to determine which markers lie near each other and are inherited together as a unit. For example, if two markers are studied and they are found to be repeatedly passed together from one generation to the next, then it is likely that they are close to each other on the same chromosome. If they are frequently passed from one generation to the next separately and independently, then they are not likely to be close together and maybe not even on the same chromosome. Making genetic maps is important for understanding the genetic locations of and distance between traits, disease genes, and specific DNA sequences. Genetic maps provide a sort of genetic compass for scientists trying to navigate their way around the genome.

Physical maps determine the actual base pair distances between the different markers on the genetic map. Knowing exactly where markers are and how far apart they are helps scientists evaluate precisely where a particular piece of DNA resides on a chromosome. Physical maps can help scientists characterize the amount of genetic material that is lost or damaged when chromosomes suffer deletions or rearrangements. Physical maps also provide a necessary tool for finding genes for specific diseases. Physical maps are like mileage charts on chromosomes.

Prior to the Human Genome Project, if a doctor wanted to find the gene responsible for a patient's medical problem, success would require finding one gene out of about 50,000 to 100,000 genes, with very little information to use as guideposts. The search would be something like being told to find Tahiti on a map of the world that had no labels, no landmarks, no reference points, no mile markers, and no addresses. What the Human Genome Project has done is to put countries, states, roads, and even addresses on that map, so that finding out where you are and how to get where you want to go is much, much easier. It's like having a bunch of big red "You Are Here" signs all over the chromosomes.

The Human Genome Project also endeavors to determine the actual nucleotide sequence of every human chromosome. Genomic sequence analysis provides the basic information that is needed to characterize genes and identify the mutations that cause disease. Once the sequence of the entire genome is known, then scientists only have to isolate particular sequences from the stockpile of information and compare typical DNA sequences to the DNA sequences found in their patients.

Sequencing the genome also provides a way to identify, analyze, and compare common structural and functional elements that can be found repeatedly throughout the genome. For example, if we know the important functional elements that one gene uses to get transcribed, and we know the sequence of the entire genome, we can search the genome for that sequence, find out how many times it occurs, which other genes use that element, and what genes might be affected if a cell loses the ability to recognize it. Alternatively, if we find a particular gene that is susceptible to a particular type of genetic rearrangement because of a certain sequence element, we can quickly find other genes that may have the same susceptibility and determine if they are in a region associated with a genetic disease. The ability to rapidly search the genome for specific sequences will expedite the identification of many genes and the analysis of many illnesses.

DNA sequence is also important for studying protein function. For example, if we learn that a particular DNA sequence is used by one protein to encode a specific function, then finding that same DNA sequence in another gene may suggest a similar capability.

In addition, the Human Genome Project plans to identify all of the individual genes of man. To do this, the nucleotide sequences that are part of the genes will be separated from the total sequence information of the genome. This initiative will result in a database containing the chromosomal address and complete nucleotide sequence of all the genes of man. This information will be available for study by doctors and scientists all over the world.

Ten years ago, if a researcher wanted to find a gene and determine its sequence, it would probably have taken many laboratory technicians a number of years to find the right region of the genome and sift through all the unrelated genetic information in the general vicinity of the gene just to zero in on what they were looking for. Ten years from now, a researcher might be able to identify the region of the genome he or she wishes to study, go to the computer, search the database, and obtain—with the touch of a key—a list of candidate genes in the right chromosomal area. The sequences of candidate genes could then be compared to the genetic sequences found in patients in an effort to identify the disease gene and determine the mutations involved in the illness.

The ability to so easily search for and identify genes will make basic science research into a variety of different medical and biological questions faster, cheaper, and more reliable. For example, scientists are only beginning to understand the molecular aspects of development, neurology, psychology, cardiology, and so many other disciplines. Having so much genetic information directly accessible will provide new tools for the study of genetic elements and their encoded proteins. These new tools will allow scientists to unravel the individual steps of pathways that must all work together to make a body work—sort of like taking a puzzle apart one piece at a time. The genome project will provide the individual puzzle pieces for analysis.

Another important aspect of the genome project is the mapping, sequencing, and characterization of the genetic information of a number of other organisms such as bacteria, yeast, fruit flies, and mice. Years of biological research has taught us that the knowledge gained from studying organisms other than man is valuable in advancing our understanding of the workings of the human body. This is because nature often uses the same biological pathways in several different organisms to accomplish the same tasks. For example, the fruit fly (*Drosophila melanogaster*) has received a great deal of attention in recent years as a model system for studying the genes involved in the construction of a body. The discovery of developmentally important genes in the fruit fly and the identification of specific genetic alterations that cause abnormalities has taught us a great deal about the process of body development.

Learning the DNA sequences of developmental genes in the fruit fly has allowed comparison of these DNA sequences with the DNA sequences of man. Comparative genetic analysis has identified of a number of developmentally important human genes. Knowing how mutations in developmental genes cause problems in the proper growth of fruit flies has led to theories about how mutations in similar genes in man might result in similar developmental abnormalities. Many of the genes found to disturb development in flies have also now been shown to disrupt the same developmental pathways in humans. Comparison of human genes with the genes of model systems such as the fly, mouse, and other organisms will continue to be a valuable research tool.

In addition to the medical applications of the Human Genome Project, the effort also promises to advance technology. Continuous technology development has been crucial to the success of the genome project. The sheer volume of the scientific discovery combined with the pace of that discovery has demanded the automation of many laboratory systems and the development of machines that do things faster, better, and cheaper. The applications of these advances in laboratory technology will be important to many fields.

The colossal amount of information that is being discovered and the extraordinarily rapid pace at which discoveries are occurring all over the world have also mandated advances in information management. As was discussed in the previous chapter, all of this data must be organized, stored, evaluated, manipulated, shared, and made available to labs and researchers everywhere.

The participation of private industry for the purposes of technology transfer is another important part of the Human Genome Project. Industry provides an outlet for the rapid application of discoveries and technologies to widespread use. Commercialization and technology transfer provide the format for moving discoveries as quickly as possible from the laboratory to the doctor's office.

Finally, the Human Genome Project has designated about 3 percent of its budget to a project called ELSI, as mentioned in Chapter 14. ELSI's goals are to investigate the ethical, legal, and social issues surrounding genetic research and testing and to encourage public and professional education and discussion. Awareness of and debate upon the issues surrounding genetic research, testing, and treatments will be crucial to the development of medically and socially responsible policies.

Among the subjects to be evaluated by ELSI is the appropriate management of genetic information with respect to privacy and confidentiality. The questions that need to be answered include who should have access to genetic information, for what reasons, and what level of patient consent is required for access. These issues are important for determining the acceptable and unacceptable uses of genetic information by patients, doctors, insurers, and employers.

Another issue that must be considered in light of modern genetic research is how to prevent social stigmatization and discrimination based on genetic information or test results. An important regulator of the social impact of genetic information will be education. An educated populace has greater protection against unrealistic claims and false expectations than an uninformed one. An educated public is also better equipped to take advantage of advances in medical care due to genetic research. In addition, education provides a basis for rational and critical public evaluation of issues and policies.

Education of medical providers such as doctors and nurses will also be crucial to the ultimate success of the Human Genome Project. If the discoveries of genetic research are to be rapidly applied to medicine for the benefit of patients, it is crucial that doctors and nurses be educated about genetics. Without proper training and education, there is always a risk for misinterpretation of test results or misinformation about genetic disease and genetic risks. Professional education will provide protection against such errors and assure appropriate application of genetic knowledge and capabilities.

Social stigmatization and genetic discrimination are not social issues only but also legal ones. The development of legislation that protects individuals against discrimination in insurance and employment based on genetic information is pending in many states and in the United States Congress. This was discussed in detail in Chapter 14. Public and professional input into the extent of protection provided by these laws will be important for the development of useful policies.

Another important ELSI concern has to do with evaluation of the psychological and cultural implications of genetic test results. Evaluation of the psychological factors relating to genetic research and testing must take into account cultural and religious differences in the way genetic information is viewed by patients, families, and society. Consideration of public perceptions about genetics will be important. Questions include how people use genetic information, how different patients react to genetic test results, what impact genetic test results have on a person's outlook and medical decisions, and how ethical, religious, and moral beliefs impact the use of medical genetics options. The answers to these questions are likely to vary depending upon cultural and religious factors as well as individual perceptions about the manageability of certain genetic diseases. As genetics moves from a largely diagnostic and predictive practice to one of treatment and prevention, the psychological factors that impact on how people accept and perceive medical genetic options are also likely to change.

ELSI also considers how to integrate genetic advances into medical practice. Questions about when and how genetic tests should be used, who will conduct such tests, and how to decide who to test and when to test them must be answered. As more genetic conditions are characterized, the opportunity for presymptomatic testing for genetic disease will grow. Genetic counseling and clinical genetics care will be important for the comprehensive management of patients and families. Evaluation of clinical genetics care and genetic counseling will be important to keep genetics professionals in step with the interests, concerns, and demands of their patients.

Research issues such as informed consent for genetic research, the ethics and practices surrounding human subjects in research, and the aspects of experimental design are also important ELSI topics. Informed consent was discussed in more detail in Chapter 14.

Finally, ELSI considers issues related to the commercialization of genetic research and technology. ELSI deals with concerns over what can and cannot be patented or copyrighted, how such material should be licensed, what constitutes trade secrets, and how to manage the availability of data and materials for the advancement of science and the benefit of patients. With regard to the commercialization of scientific data and technology, it is important that the scientific advances are rapidly moved into the public and commercial sectors so that the benefit to doctors, patients, and their families is maximized. But at the same time, companies and researchers have concerns over protection of their inventions, discoveries, and data. These different concerns must be balanced in a responsible manner that optimizes the application of genetic information and methods to medical practice. Public and professional discussion of these and many other issues is likely to continue for years to come.

For more information on the Human Genome Project, visit your library, bookstore, or these Internet sites:

- The National Human Genome Research Institute
  (http://www.nhgri.nih.gov)
- The Human Genome Project
  (http://www.ornl.gov/TechResources/Human_Genome/tko/index.htm)
- The Human Genome Organization
  (http://www.gene.ucl.ac.uk/hugo/)

CHAPTER TWENTY-TWO

Gene Therapy and Other Treatments for Genetic Disease

Advances in our understanding of how genetic defects cause disease are bringing about greater promise for effective treatment. Some genetic diseases are treatable using methods that replace missing but necessary metabolic products or that help in the removal of harmful metabolites that build up due to enzyme defects. A good example is the autosomal recessive disorder phenylketonuria, or PKU. As we have learned in previous chapters, PKU is caused by a deficiency of an enzyme, phenylalanine hydroxylase. The absence of the enzyme causes the accumulation of the amino acid phenylalanine in the tissues of the affected individual. The deficiency of the enzyme together with the accumulation of phenylalanine can result in profound mental retardation in affected individuals. Biochemical understanding of the disorder has provided simple and effective dietary intervention. Affected individuals are put on strictly controlled diets, limiting their intake of phenylalanine. Adherence to the prescribed diet alleviates the buildup of phenylalanine and dramatically reduces the risk of mental impairment in PKU patients.

Another autosomal recessive disease that can be effectively treated by a similar approach is galactosemia. Dietary intervention to control the intake of galactose generally alleviates the most devastating symptoms of the disease.

Some genetic diseases are treatable by replacement therapies where the missing or deficient enzyme or compound is provided. For example, Gaucher disease is an autosomal recessive enzyme deficiency seen most frequently in individuals of Ashkenazi Jewish descent. Currently, enzyme replacement therapy allows patients to acquire the missing enzyme, often significantly reducing symptoms. Another example of a replacement therapy is

173

biotinidase deficiency, in which doctors can provide patients with biotin and thereby alleviate many if not all of the symptoms of the disease.

Genetic diseases for which dietary restriction and enzyme or factor replacement approaches are not effective present a more complex therapeutic challenge. Many such disorders cannot be effectively managed at the present time. Some of these diseases are the target of gene therapy research. Gene therapy is also sometimes referred to as gene transfer therapy. Some nongenetic disorders and other types of medical problems are also the subject of gene therapy research. Disorders for which gene therapy is currently being considered include CF, alpha-1 antitrypsin deficiency, DMD, cancer, AIDS, atherosclerosis, spinal cord injury, and many others.

Gene therapy methods differ from the more conventional treatment approaches described above because gene therapy is aimed at removal of the cause of a disease, not just alleviation of the symptoms. The goal of gene therapy is to deliver genes rather than proteins, enzymes, or drugs. The theory is that the delivered genes, when inside cells and transcribed into RNA, will provide the missing protein or evoke the desired cellular response. The result will be the removal of the cause and the complete relief of the symptoms of a disorder.

In its simplest forms, gene therapy would be used for the treatment of diseases caused by missing or nonfunctional proteins such as enzyme deficiencies or the absence of structural or regulatory proteins. For disorders such as CF, Gaucher disease, alpha-1 antitrypsin deficiency, or hemophilia that are caused by the absence of a particular protein function, the idea behind gene therapy is to provide cells with the missing protein or enzyme function by providing a working copy of the gene that has suffered a mutation. Theoretically, once in place, the delivered gene will be expressed and will rescue the cells—and the patient—from the effects of the disease.

In its more complex forms, it is hoped that gene therapy can provide proteins or enzymes to eliminate an undesired cellular function. For example, for the gene therapy of cancer, the goal is to provide a protein that can either render cancer cells susceptible to cytotoxic (cell killing) drugs or in some other way curb the uncontrolled cell divisions characteristic of cancer cells.

In these cases, gene therapy would be directed toward the cancer cells specifically. After the new gene is delivered, cell death could be specifically induced either by the administration of drugs that would kill the cells carrying the new gene or by some internal mechanism resulting from the action of the delivered gene. Antiviral gene therapy, for diseases such as AIDS, is likely to be geared either toward making infected cells susceptible to highly efficient destruction by cytotoxic drugs or toward preventing the infection, replication, and spread of the virus. For spinal cord injury and other similar problems, gene therapy is likely to be geared toward stimulating the cells of the body to grow and repair damaged organs or tissues.

For genetic diseases in which gene mutations result in a protein that has either gained a new function or interferes with other proteins, more complex approaches may be required. For these types of mutations, gene therapy would have to deliver a gene that would produce an RNA or protein to inhibit the gained function. It is not yet clear how effective such treatments might be.

On paper, gene therapy looks easy. Just give a patient a gene and solve everybody's problems. But in reality, gene therapy is very challenging. The major challenges facing gene therapy researchers include: how to deliver genes to cells, how to deliver those genes to the right cells, how to assure that the gene is used properly by cells, how to make the gene work for long periods of time, and how to assure that the treatment is safe for the patient and for others.

The first thing gene therapy researchers must consider is how to get a gene into a cell. If a gene cannot get into a cell, there is no way that gene therapy can work. Much of the current gene therapy research is focused on the development of viruses that can be used as vectors, or delivery systems, to carry genes into cells.

Viruses are tiny organisms that are made up of a protein shell or coat that encases the genetic material of the virus, either DNA or RNA. In nature, viruses infect cells, deliver their genes into cells, and use the cell's machinery to replicate their DNA or RNA and make proteins. These processes result in the manufacture of new viruses for further infection of new cells.

In gene therapy research, candidate viruses are manipulated in the laboratory to carry human genes instead of viral genes. With human genes instead of viral genes packaged into the virus protein shell, the viruses essentially are tricked into delivering human genes to target cells. In this way, when the virus infects a cell, it is unable to make virus proteins because it lacks virus genes. The hope is that, once inside a cell, the virus will express the human gene and that the proper protein will be made. The goal is to have the protein work in the cell and replace the missing function, resulting in relief of disease symptoms.

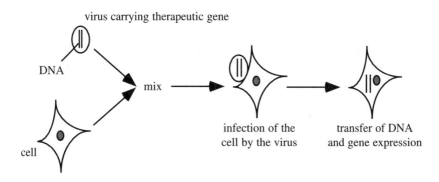

FIGURE 22.1   A diagram of how gene therapy might be performed using a virus as the vector for introducing genes into a target cell. The gene of interest is introduced into a laboratory-made virus. The virus is then allowed to infect a target cell that needs the gene carried by the virus. Once inside the target cell, the cell should begin to express the gene and provide a protein therapeutic to the disease.

There are also a variety of nonviral gene delivery systems that have been considered as possible vectors for gene transfer experiments. Liposomes, for example, are tiny particles that are made up of DNA surrounded by a membrane similar to a cell membrane. The idea is to fuse the liposome with a target cell to introduce the DNA. Future research will be needed to clarify the most efficient uses for the different types of gene transfer vectors.

Getting a gene to the right place in the body is the next challenge of gene therapy. Getting a gene to the wrong place is not likely to help much, unless it produces a protein that can move freely from cell to cell or acts on a substance that moves freely from cell to cell. For example, if one wants to perform gene therapy for CF, one needs to consider the symptoms of CF, the protein deficiency that causes CF, and the function of that protein.

CF is caused by mutations in the gene for a protein called the cystic fibrosis transmembrane conductance regulator (CFTR). The CFTR protein embeds itself in the cell membrane that surrounds certain cells. It is believed to be involved in the transport of molecules such as chloride across the cell membrane. The goal for CF gene therapy will be to deliver a functional copy of the CFTR gene to cells that show the greatest impairment due to deficiency of the protein. Since the most devastating, life threatening symptoms of CF involve respiratory difficulties, lung cells are considered to be the primary target for CF gene therapy. The challenge for CF gene therapy will be to develop a vector system that can ensure efficient delivery of the CFTR gene to a large number of lung cells.

Current ideas about gene therapy for CF involve using modified viruses that can be inhaled by patients or somehow otherwise delivered to the cells lining the airway. The hope is that the delivered virus particles will efficiently infect lung and airway cells. If these virus particles carry the CFTR gene instead of viral genes, then they may be an effective means to deliver the CFTR gene to lung cells. If the CFTR protein is expressed after infection, then proper respiratory function may be restored, alleviating the most devastating symptoms of CF.

Herein lies the next challenge of gene therapy: Once a gene is delivered to the proper cells, it must get expressed. If a gene is transferred into a cell but is not expressed, there is not going to be any benefit from the procedure. A great deal of gene therapy research is centered around making sure that, along with the gene, efficient promoter and RNA processing signals are also transferred. We learned about these control elements in Chapter 5. These control signals may not be the same for every gene. Genetic research focused on the identification of transcription signals needed for optimum expression of transferred genes is necessary to assure successful gene therapy.

Another concern for gene therapy is to get genes expressed for long periods of time. It is great if a gene can get into a cell and get expressed, but if it is only expressed for a few days or weeks, the symptoms of the disease are likely to recur, and the patients will not be any better off than they were before the procedure. In addition, the treatment would have to be repeated frequently. One obstacle to long-term expression of genes in gene therapy is the transient nature of some viruses. If the viruses carry the therapeutic gene to cells but do not hang around very long, then the therapeutic gene will go with them. If the therapeutic gene goes with them, then so does the treatment. In the case of short-term virus persistence, one alternative might be repeated treatment with the virus. While this would be less convenient than a one-shot cure, it may be the only option in some cases.

The introduction of new proteins into cells faces yet another challenge from the immune system. If the patient develops an immune response to the protein made by the delivered gene, then the immune system of the patient might develop antibodies or T cells to destroy the protein or the cells making the protein. Alternatively, the patient could develop an immune response to the viral vector used to deliver the gene. If this occurs, then the therapeutic protein might be removed from the patient's system, symptoms could recur, and the patient may be back to being sick again.

In actuality though, the patient may be even worse off than before because subsequent treatments might not be effective if the immune system now recognizes the transferred protein or the virus used to carry the gene into cells. If this happens, the immune response could interfere with future treatments. Research into how much of a problem this will be and how to reduce or eliminate interference from the immune system may be necessary before some forms of gene therapy can achieve their maximum effectiveness.

A final major consideration of gene therapy is safety. If viruses are used in gene therapy, scientists must be certain that they are not creating some new virus—one that is capable of spreading an infection. To introduce a new virus into the environment could be dangerous. In theory, viruses that do not carry viral genes cannot cause infection in the traditional sense. So by deleting viral genes from a gene therapy virus, the viruses are disabled and they cannot make more viruses. If the virus cannot direct the manufacture of more viruses, it cannot spread infection. As such, the gene therapy viruses are purposefully designed to be effective for only a single infection of a target cell and for delivery of the intended human genes. In practice, all gene therapy viruses will have to be tested to assure this level of safety before they can be implemented in large numbers of patients.

Another safety concern for gene therapy is the effect that the introduction of a virus has on a cell. Scientists must be sure that the introduced virus does not induce new cellular mutations that could result in some other medical problem or cause some undesired side effect. The risk of these problems with different types of viruses will need to be carefully evaluated before virus-based gene therapy vectors can be widely used.

Much of the controversy surrounding gene therapy has been over the alteration of the genetic makeup of human beings. This is because some of the viruses under consideration actually insert their genetic material into the genome of the cell that they infect. These viruses are called "retroviruses."

The result of infection of a cell with a retrovirus is that the genes carried into the cell by the retrovirus are permanently inserted into the genetic material of the cell. The viral genetic material remains in the genetic material of the cell and its descendants for all future cell divisions.

This feature is what makes a retrovirus such an attractive vector for gene therapy. Infection of a cell by a retrovirus carrying a therapeutic gene could theoretically be permanent and, if efficient, alleviate the need for additional treatments. However, if by chance the virus interrupts another gene when it sits down in the cell's genome, then the function of that gene may be impaired for the rest of that cell's and its daughter cells' lives. If this is a crucial gene for some needed function, the gene therapy procedure might effectively solve one problem but cause another.

To avoid this, gene therapy using retroviruses is performed on a large number of cells, not just on one cell. If a number of cells are treated and one of the cells has an important function interrupted, then the other treated cells will be around to take up the slack. It is unlikely that the same function would be impaired in all cells treated.

There is also the risk that a transferred gene might sit down in a gene that can lead to cancer. Since cancer is generally caused by a cascade of multiple mutations, as discussed in Chapter 12, the likelihood that this might happen is unknown in any given patient. Future research and gene therapy trials will have to address these risks.

An extra measure of safety is provided by performing gene therapy on somatic cells only. Somatic cell gene therapy would not involve treatment of germ cells and therefore would not affect future generations. In fact, current efforts at gene therapy are aimed only at somatic cells, cells not destined to become sperm or eggs. Therefore, just like drug therapies, somatic cell gene therapy is a treatment for the affected individual only. Children of the patient would still be at risk for inheriting the genetic deficiencies that caused the disease.

Germ line gene therapy, an approach that delivers genes to sperm or eggs, is highly controversial because of its potential effect on future generations. Germ line gene therapy could potentially eliminate disease in future generations by repairing the original genetic defect in germ cells. However, germ line gene therapy carries an unknown level of risk. For example, if a gene that was transferred in the course of gene therapy inadvertently interrupted another gene, the child could be cured of one problem but born affected with a different genetic problem. The present viral methods of gene transfer have unknown risks for human embryos and fetuses because they do not guarantee insertion of the transferred genes into specific sites. As a result, germ line gene therapy is not being considered for application to humans at this time.

However, if scientists could figure out how to make sure that a transferred gene goes into the cell's genome at the same spot as the already mutated gene, then the safety of germ line gene therapy procedures might be dramatically increased. Additional research is required before these methods could be applied to humans.

Somatic cell gene therapy clinical trials are currently under way for a number of genetic diseases and proposed for a number of others. Frequently, patients can be enrolled in research protocols. Your doctor or geneticist may be able to help you identify the site of gene therapy clinical trials for a genetic disease you are concerned about.

Patients and families may also be able to discover the institutions conducting clinical trials themselves. Sources such as the scientific literature, newspapers, television, support groups, and research foundations can provide information on clinical trials. In addition, the Internet sites for the National Institutes of Health (http://www.nih.gov/health), the National Cancer Institute (http://cancertrials.nci.nih.gov), and Mediconsult (http://www.mediconsult.com) have information about ongoing clinical trials of many kinds, not just gene therapy. These and other information resources are discussed in more detail in Chapters 26-28.

CHAPTER TWENTY-THREE

Cloning

Cloning is a method for creating an exact copy of something. As we discussed in Chapter 19, the isolation and duplication of genes or small portions of DNA containing genes is one type of cloning. In this type of cloning, the isolated DNA is inserted into the genetic material of a bacteria, virus, or yeast. Placing a piece of human DNA into a bacteria, virus, or yeast allows for rapid and efficient production of millions of copies of the sequence. This facilitates characterization of and experimentation with the DNA segment.

The cloning of genes also allows the development of vectors for gene therapy, as discussed in the previous chapter. These types of cloning—that is, the cloning of genes—do not involve the duplication of whole animals. The cloning of genes is crucial to the continued success of human genetic research and testing and to the eventual development of effective treatments for people with illnesses of all kinds.

For therapeutic applications, cloning of genes provides a safe source of proteins to treat illness. As discussed in Chapter 19, providing patients with a protein that they are missing because of mutations in a gene may alleviate the symptoms of many genetic diseases. Cloned proteins such as human growth hormone and insulin have been successfully used to treat short stature and diabetes, respectively.

Another application for gene cloning is vaccine development through the cloning of genes for bacterial and viral proteins. Cloning for vaccine development can provide for the rapid, safe, and abundant production of viral proteins. Cloned proteins can be administered to patients for the purpose of evoking an immune response. Vaccines that are developed using cloned proteins are often called recombinant vaccines. This approach has already been used to develop vaccines for Hepatitis B and will certainly continue to be used in the future.

Another type of cloning involves the duplication of whole cells for research or therapeutic purposes. Some of the many applications for this type of cloning include growing populations of cells with a specific genetic defect to study the effects of gene mutations; growing populations of cells with a specific genetic defect to test the effectiveness of gene therapy and other types of treatments; growing an individual's own cells for repair of organs and tissues after illness, infection, or injury; and development of organs and tissues compatible with a variety of immune systems. The first two applications have the ability to rapidly advance medical knowledge and the treatment of disease. The latter two have the potential to provide limitless sources of immunologically compatible donor organs for transplant, donor organs that could shorten or eliminate transplant waiting lists and reduce the complications of graft versus host disease.

One application of cell cloning technology that has received a great deal of attention in recent weeks is that of human stem cell research. Stem cells are cells that are at an early stage of development: cells that have the potential to develop into many different cell types. The use of human stem cells to repair and regenerate damaged organs and tissues is actively being studied. The idea is that stem cells could be used to replace damaged cells in a variety of human tissues. The potential of this research for the treatment of human disease is immense. However, the sources of these cells, embryonic or fetal, are quite controversial and currently a matter of much public debate.

Another application for tissue cloning includes the production of populations of cells such as bone marrow that produce therapeutic compounds for the treatment of genetic disease. Theoretically, there are a number of applications of this type of technology. For example, in patients with hemophilia who lack a protein necessary for proper clotting of the blood, transplants using specifically cloned bone marrow might be able to provide the missing protein and solve the bleeding problems experienced by these patients.

Another type of cloning, the cloning of animals, got a great deal of media attention at the time that the Scottish sheep, Dolly, was cloned in 1996. Dolly was the first mammal reportedly cloned from the cells of an adult mammal. In the experiment, a single mammary cell from an adult sheep was isolated and fused with the egg cell from another sheep, an egg cell that had its nucleus removed (see the diagram in Figure 23.1 on the next page). The removal of the nucleus of the egg eliminated most of the genetic contribution of the egg to the future animal and replaced it with the genetic contribution from the donor mammary cell of the adult sheep.

The media coverage that resulted from the cloning of Dolly sparked an important public debate over cloning technology and how it should be used. More recent reports of the cloning of cattle and mice have renewed the discussion, making it clear that this technology is not going to disappear.

The public discussion about cloning technology so far has focused largely on the possibility of cloning human beings. The societal debate over the applications of cloning technology is important because there are certain applications of this technology that are beneficial and there are others that are controversial. Ultimately, the legislation adopted to regulate the technology must be well thought out and carefully written so that the potentially beneficial applications of cloning technology can be spared while the objectionable applications can be prohibited.

In consideration of the technological aspects of cloning and how to legislate them, the variety of potential applications must be considered. There are a number of examples that have already been presented in this chapter. For example, the cloning of genes and cells has been going on for years and is crucial to the continued development of medical science. These applications do not involve the cloning of entire animals and would not need to be regulated or prohibited to avoid the creation of a human child by cloning. The following list includes other potential applications of cloning technology.

- The development of animals such as cattle, sheep, or goats that produce therapeutic human proteins in their milk. Consider a herd of cattle that might be produced to make clotting factors in their milk for the safe and effective treatment of hemophilia. Such sources

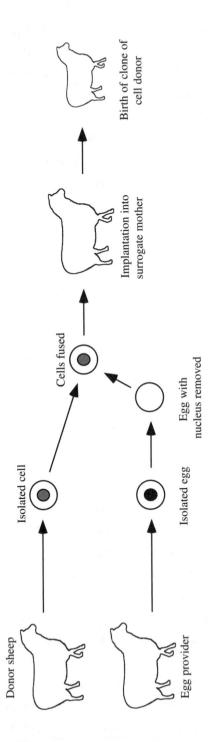

FIGURE 23.1 Diagram of the technique that was used to create Dolly. In the cloning of Dolly, a process called somatic cell nuclear transfer was used. Somatic cell nuclear transfer involves several steps. The first step is the removal of a nucleus from a sheep's egg cell. This enucleated egg is then fused with a mammary cell isolated from an adult sheep. The resulting embryo is transplanted into a surrogate mother sheep for gestation. In this case, the somatic cell nuclear transfer procedure resulted in the birth of the lamb Dolly. Theoretically, the lamb carries the nucleus and therefore the chromosomal genetic material of the donor adult sheep and is essentially an identical twin to that adult sheep—a twin that was born many years later.

could be a simple and effective way to produce mass quantities of the therapeutic protein.

- The development of high-yield agricultural crops that are resistant to pests or disease. Development of such crops might increase crop yield, providing a larger food supply while also decreasing the need for chemical pesticides or fertilizers.

- The cloning of endangered species in times of crisis and when captive breeding programs are failing. Cloning of animals in this context could help sustain a species through the temporary loss of habitat or while breeding programs are being established.

- The production of genetically identical animals for biomedical research. Genetically identical animals in research are useful because they minimize variability in genetic factors that can influence disease expression and measurement of treatment effectiveness. Removing the genetic variables from experiments can accelerate research by providing a uniform test system in which controlled variables can be modulated.

Most of the legislation that has been proposed has been geared toward prohibiting the creation of a human child by cloning. Many people have put forth a variety of social, religious, moral, and ethical reasons why the cloning of a human being would be objectionable. Many of these reasons are valid and must be considered in the context of developing legislation.

Social, religious, and moral arguments notwithstanding, many scientists have provided purely scientific reasons to prohibit the cloning of human beings at the present time—safety being the most prominent. Seldom mentioned is the number of times Dolly was attempted before success was achieved. Twenty-nine embryos resulted from 277 cell/egg fusions and only one lamb was born. That is a lot of lost embryos and fetuses. Clearly, the method is neither effective nor safe enough to consider for application to human fetuses at the present time. In fact, considering the great expense and effort and the advanced technology involved in creating just a single animal, it is likely that it will be some time before this technology will have any widespread application, even in animals. It is currently much cheaper and easier to breed animals of desired genotypes and phenotypes than it is to clone them. After all, agriculture, farming, and the domestication and selective breeding of plants and animals has been going on for thousands of years without the application of molecular genetic science.

Another safety concern involves the correct expression of genes. During the growth and development of an animal, certain genes are switched on and off as they are needed to build a body. Most of the genes that worked early in the development of that adult sheep had probably long since been switched off in the donor mammary cell. When the donor cell was fused with the egg to make Dolly, all those early developmental genes had to get switched back on in order to allow the embryo to grow into a whole, live-born sheep. Also, remember that Dolly is female, because the donor sheep was female. As such, the donor mammary cell had one X chromosome that was inactivated.

Herein lies the great breakthrough in the cloning of Dolly: Never before has such an extensive attempt to reactivate this many genes at once been successful in a mammal. Until Dolly was cloned, there was no proof that such a large-scale reactivation of developmental genes could even occur in a complex organism such as a mammal.

And what about X inactivation? Dolly is a female, so each of her cells has one active and one inactive X chromosome. In the donor cell that was used to make Dolly, one of the X chromosomes was inactive. Does Dolly have only one X chromosome active in all of her cells or was the inactive X switched back on in the embryo so that random X inactivation could proceed normally? Would the same thing happen in a human embryo? If Dolly never reactivated the donor's inactive X chromosome, all her cells would express just one X chromosome. Could she—and other clones—be susceptible to genetic disease if the active X in the donor cell carries an unrecognized gene with a mutation?

For human cloning, the reactivation of developmental genes whether or not on the X chromosome is a complex question. Clearly, enough genes were reactivated to result in at least one live-born sheep, but there is no evidence as to whether reactivation of every gene necessary to produce a healthy, normal human being can be guaranteed. Are 100 percent of the genes switched back on? Or are some genes permanently inactivated? Is 97 percent a more realistic approximation?

Remember, twenty-nine implanted embryos resulted in only one live birth. What was the cause of those losses? Why were all those embryos and fetuses not viable? Did it have something to do with the conditions of the cell culture in the laboratory? Or was it incomplete reactivation of genes? Were there lethal mutations in the DNA of the donor cells? Would mental retardation in a human clone be more likely than in a human child produced by sexual reproduction? What about developmental abnormalities? No one knows, which illustrates why it is not appropriate at this time to attempt this technology on humans.

One final safety concern for cloning of a human being is the accumulation of genetic damage. Genetic damage and DNA base substitutions are now recognized as a normal part of the aging process. As a result, Dolly has started out with the genetic damage of an adult. It is not yet clear how inheriting a lifetime's accumulation of somatic mutations will affect Dolly. She may not be significantly affected. Or she may live a shorter-than-normal life span. She may be at risk for certain genetic diseases at an earlier age than usual. No one yet knows. And suppose there were some devastating mutation in that one cell that was used as a donor, could that result in unpredictable genetic disease in the clone? This uncertainty is a final reason why it would not be appropriate to consider the application of this technology to humans at this time.

For research purposes however, Dolly's birth is significant. Dolly's birth provides evidence that genes can be reactivated after a cell passes through a certain developmental phase. This is important information because it suggests that this might be accomplished on a cellular scale solely for the treatment of disease. For example, consider the development of humans. Early in development, there is an active human gene that encodes a fetal form of the protein hemoglobin, the protein that carries oxygen in the blood. Later in development, the gene for the fetal form of hemoglobin gets switched off and the gene for the adult form of hemoglobin gets switched on. In patients with β-thalassemia, who lack a working gene for the adult hemoglobin protein, their blood is not able to carry oxygen efficiently. This can result in very serious illness. However, if doctors could effectively and permanently reactivate that fetal hemoglobin gene, they might be able to alleviate many of the symptoms in these patients by providing a working, albeit fetal, hemoglobin molecule.

This is only one potential application of the ability to reactivate individual genes or small sets of genes. Learning how to reactivate certain genes could be applied to the treatment of many genetic diseases and nongenetic injuries such as spinal cord damage from trauma, liver damage from viral infections or cancer, or heart damage after a heart attack. Being able to reactivate genes in these tissues might lead to regenerative repair of damaged organs and reacquisition of lost functions. None of these potential applications would involve the creation of a human child through cloning, but instead would involve experimentation on cells.

Legislation is under development worldwide that would prohibit the application of this technology to the creation of a human child. At the present time, this is a prudent course of action, endorsed by scientific, religious, and political groups alike. But as described here, the technology used in these types of experiments could be used for a variety of important medical and biological purposes, none of which would involve the creation of a human child by cloning. These beneficial applications of the technology must be considered when writing legislation that would regulate the technology's use. We must prohibit the application of the technology to certain objectionable purposes, but we must be careful not to restrict science in such a way as to prevent beneficial uses of the technology.

Throughout history, mankind has been challenged to balance the possible benefits against the potential for misuse of many technologies, and genetic science is no different. A meaningful discussion between science and an educated public will be necessary to adopt a collective understanding of how we as a society wish these new technologies to be applied for the good of man and nature.

CHAPTER TWENTY-FOUR

The Practitioners of Medical Genetics

Clinical Geneticists

Clinical geneticists are medical doctors, holding M.D. degrees. Clinical geneticists have special training and expertise in the diagnosis and treatment of genetic disease and see patients in a clinical setting such as a doctor's office. They are an excellent resource for individuals and families concerned about the diagnosis of genetic disease in a child or an adult.

Many clinical geneticists are also specialists in other areas of medicine such as Pediatrics, Neurology, Ophthalmology, or Obstetrics and Gynecology (Ob/Gyn). They may be associated with a medical school or hospital or may practice independently. Clinical geneticists who have successfully completed the required training and qualifying examinations are certified by the American Board of Medical Genetics.

Genetic Counselors

Genetic counselors are highly trained professionals who can provide patients with information, counseling, and referrals regarding genetic disease, genetic testing, recurrence risk, and treatment options. Genetic counselors generally have master's degrees in genetic counseling, but some genetic counselors have Ph.D. degrees. Genetic counselors are not physicians, but often work in conjunction with physicians, clinics, and laboratories to help in communicating genetic risks, testing options, test results, reproductive options, and many other aspects of genetics to patients. Genetic counselors are an excellent resource for families or individuals concerned about a genetic disease and interested in information and assistance. Genetic counselors who have successfully completed the required training and qualifying examinations are certified by the American Board of Genetic Counseling.

Clinical Laboratory Geneticists

Laboratory geneticists are either medical doctors with M.D. degrees or laboratory-trained doctors carrying Ph.D. degrees. Some laboratory geneticists hold both degrees. Laboratory geneticists have special training and expertise in human genetics and in the biochemical or molecular aspects of genetic disease.

The three main specialties in laboratory genetics are cytogenetics, the study of the chromosomal makeup of cells; molecular genetics, the study of DNA and genes; and biochemical genetics, the study of the biochemical content and metabolism of cells. Many laboratory geneticists are associated with medical schools and hospitals, and many are associated with private diagnostic laboratories or companies. Clinical Cytogeneticists, Clinical Biochemical Geneticists, and Clinical Molecular Geneticists who have successfully completed the required training and qualifying examinations are certified by the American Board of Medical Genetics.

Research Geneticists

Research scientists from many fields have become involved in genetic research through their work. Research scientists who head laboratories generally hold Ph.D. degrees, but some may hold M.D. degrees or both Ph.D. and M.D. degrees. Research geneticists are generally involved in basic scientific inquiry and in discovery of the causes, effects, and possible treatments of genetic disease. It is usually in the laboratory that the basic knowledge of a genetic disease is gained and advances in treatment are developed.

Sometimes patients can be enrolled in research projects or in clinical trials. Genetic counselors and clinical geneticists can often inform patients about ongoing research programs that are enrolling patients. Support groups, research foundations, and the scientific literature are other potential sources of information about research for genetic diseases and clinical trials. These resources will be discussed in more detail in Chapters 26–28.

CHAPTER TWENTY-FIVE

How to Find Genetics Professionals in Your Area

If you do not have a geneticist already, finding one may seem like a daunting task, particularly if you are in a new city or town. Here is some advice about how to find these professionals in your area.

Your Current Physicians

Contact your family physician or, in the case of a child, your child's Pediatrician. Your physician may be able to help with your questions and concerns, especially if he or she has had training and experience in testing for or treating the genetic disease about which you are concerned.

If your physician or Pediatrician cannot help, Obstetrics/Gynecology and Perinatology specialists are often good resources for genetic information, treatment, and/or referrals. When talking to a doctor for the first time about genetics, it is important to ask several questions. These include asking about the disease with which you are concerned and its inheritance, your doctor's training and experience in genetics, the status of insurance/employment protection laws in your state with regard to genetic information, what costs your medical insurance will cover, and how the privacy and protection of your medical genetic records will be handled by your doctor.

Genetics Specialists

Many times, patients will find that they know as much about their genetic concerns as their physician does, especially if their physician is not a specialist in genetics. If this is the case, you are likely to feel that you need more information than your physician can provide. If you feel that you would like to see a certified geneticist, you may either wish to ask your physician specifically for a referral to a clinical geneticist or genetic counselor or try finding one on your own.

Genetics professionals will be able to provide detailed information about the disease with which you are concerned as well as the most recent advances in diagnosis and treatment and privacy/anti-discrimination laws. To find a genetics professional yourself, try using a combination of the following methods.

- Contact the Department of Genetics at a nearby medical school or children's hospital. Many medical schools and children's hospitals now have a genetics department or at least a program geared toward education and clinical service in genetics. Medical schools and children's hospitals with genetics programs can help by providing information and directing you to individuals who can schedule appointments with clinical geneticists and/or genetics counselors.

- Contact the National Society of Genetic Counselors on the Internet at http://www.nsgc.org or by mail at Dept. P, 233 Canterbury Drive, Wallingford, PA 19086. This organization can provide information about genetic counseling in general and about genetic counselors in your area. Genetic counselors are an excellent resource for locating clinical geneticists in your area.

- Many areas of the country now have physician referral companies or other similar services that advertise in the media. These information services may be able to provide referrals to genetics specialists.

- In addition, many hospitals and medical schools also operate their own physician referral services. Calling the physician referral offices of nearby institutions may be useful in identifying clinical geneticists or genetic counselors and scheduling appointments.

Organizations and Support Groups

If you have concerns about a particular genetic disease, you may find it useful to identify a national or local research, treatment, or support group for that disease. Such organizations include the Muscular Dystrophy Association, the March of Dimes, the American Cancer Society, the National Marfan Foundation, the Cystic Fibrosis Foundation, and many others.

You may also find assistance through organizational groups such as the Alliance of Genetic Support Groups, the March of Dimes, or the Council of Regional Networks for Genetic Services. Groups such as these provide a kind of clearinghouse for genetic disease societies, support groups, genetic counselors, and physicians. They are often able to help locate physicians or specific support groups in your area.

Specific support groups may be able to help by providing information, referrals to genetics professionals, and addresses of additional assistance and support groups in your area. A brief list of some of these organizations is provided in Chapters 26 and 27.

Other Resources

You may find your local yellow pages to be a helpful resource. In the yellow pages, look under the possible headings: Physician Referral or Physicians Referral and Information Services; Physicians (remember to also look under subheadings such as Genetics, Pediatrics, Ob/Gyn, Neurologists, or other specialties as your concerns may warrant); Clinics—Medical; Medical Schools; Hospitals; Laboratories (Medical or Clinical); or Foundations—Educational, Philanthropic, Research, etc. Remember, depending on how your phone books are organized, you may need to look under several headings in the yellow pages or phone book to find the information you need.

Finally, if you have access to the Internet, you may find it a useful resource for locating a genetics professional or genetics resources in your area. Try one of these sites:

- The Council of Regional Networks for Genetic Services, also known as CORN (http://www.cc.emory.edu/PEDIATRICS/corn/corn.htm—Click on the "contact information" button.)

- March of Dimes Birth Defects Foundation
  (http://www.modimes.org)
- National Society of Genetic Counselors
  (http:.//www.nsgc.org)
- The Genetics Professional Home Page/Genetics Education Center
  (http://www.kumc.edu/gec/prof/genecntr.html)

Be persistent. Especially if you live in an isolated or rural area, you may need to make a number of calls to several sources to find the professionals you want. The information and assistance you want is out there, but be prepared to work to find it.

CHAPTER TWENTY-SIX

Genetics Societies, Support Groups, and Foundations

There are many societies, support groups, and associations that can provide information about the symptoms, diagnosis, and treatment of specific genetic diseases. These groups can also provide information on medical, social, and educational resources in your area. The names and phone numbers of many support groups or research or medical foundations may be obtained through your doctor or genetics professional. You may also be able to find such resources through the phone book or other sources as described in the previous chapter.

For your convenience, this chapter includes the addresses and phone numbers of a few such organizations in the United States. This is in no way a complete list of the hundreds of groups in the U. S., but is rather a list of resources for some of the more commonly diagnosed genetic diseases. The addresses of these groups, obtained through the Internet, are naturally subject to change.

These addresses were found using two approaches that may be useful if you are searching for an organization not listed here. First, use one of the Internet search engines such as Netscape, Lycos, Yahoo!, or Infoseek. Type in the name of the disease about which you are interested, run the search, and see what comes up. Often, you will find the names of organizations this way. Second, if you already know the name of the support group or organization you are looking for, use the name of the organization as the search term in the Internet search. This will often lead you to the Internet home page of the group you seek.

Some groups, especially those that do not have Web sites, may be harder to find. So if the disease for which you have a concern is not listed here, if you do not have access to the Internet, or if neither of the above Internet search approaches works, there are other options to try. You may be able to find the addresses and phone numbers of helpful groups through general groups such as The Alliance of Genetic Support Groups, the March of Dimes, the Council of Regional Networks for Genetic Services, the National Society of Genetic Counselors, or one of the other general resources listed in this chapter. Some of these groups run a sort of clearinghouse listing for genetic societies and support groups. Others can help with physician referrals. Contact one or more of these groups and ask about the particular disease with which you are concerned. Tell them the city and state in which you live. See if they can provide you with a specific resource close to where you live.

If that does not work, try following the advice in the previous chapter on finding a genetics professional in your area. Contact with such individuals can help you find the resources you want.

The following list is not an endorsement of any group nor is it an assurance of the accuracy of any information you might obtain. Always double check all information with your physician or genetics professional to assure its accuracy and relevance to your medical concerns. If you have access to the Internet, the Web site addresses for most of the organizations listed below are provided in the next chapter.

General Resources

Alliance of Genetic Support Groups

> 4301 Connecticut Avenue NW, Suite 404
> Washington, DC 20008-2304
> phone 202-966-5557; toll free 800-336-GENE or 800-336-4363
> fax 202-966-8553

The Council of Regional Networks for Genetic Services (CORN)

> phone 404-727-4549

March of Dimes Birth Defects Foundation

>1275 Mamaroneck Avenue
>
>White Plains, NY 10605
>
>phone 914-428-7100; toll free 888-MODIMES or 888-663-4637

This is the national office. You may also wish to try to locate a local or regional office.

Med Help International

>Suite 130, Box 188, 6300 North Wickham Road
>
>Melbourne, FL 32940
>
>phone 407-253-9048

National Foundation for Jewish Genetic Diseases, Inc.

>250 Park Ave., Suite 1000
>
>New York, NY 10017
>
>phone 212-371-1030

National Organization for Rare Disorders, Inc. (NORD)

>P. O. Box 8923
>
>New Fairfield, CT 06812-8923
>
>phone 203-746-6518; toll free 800-999-6673
>
>fax 203-746-6481

National Society of Genetic Counselors

>Dept. P, 233 Canterbury Drive
>
>Wallingford, PA, 19086-6617
>
>phone 610-872-7608

United Way Helpline

>(Denver) phone 303-433-8900

Specific Groups

Keep in mind that there are hundreds of different support groups nationwide and many more worldwide. This is only a short list. Also, there may be more than one organization for a particular disorder, and you may wish to seek assistance from more than one group.

Achondroplasia

Little People of America
>P.O. Box 9897
>
>Washington, DC 20016
>
>phone toll free 888-LPA-2001 or 888-572-2001

Alpha-1 Antitrypsin Deficiency:

Alpha-1 National Association
>4220 Old Shakopee Road, Suite 101
>
>Minneapolis, MN 55437-2974
>
>phone 612-703-9979
>
>fax 612-885-0133

Angelman Syndrome:

Angelman Syndrome Foundation, USA
>P.O. Box 12437
>
>Gainesville, FL 32604
>
>phone toll free 800-IF-ANGEL or 800-432-6435
>
>fax 212-779-7728

Ataxias:

National Ataxia Foundation
There are two apparently separate organizations with this same name. One is at:
>2600 Fernbrook Lane, Suite 119
>
>Minneapolis, MN 55447
>
>phone 612-553-0020
>
>fax 612-553-0167

The other is located at:
>750 Twelve Oaks Center, 15550 Wayzata Blvd.
>
>Wayzata, MN 55391
>
>phone 612-473-7666
>
>fax 612-473-9289

Blood Disorders: *(see also Hemophilia)*
Cooley Anemia Foundation, Inc.
>129-09 26th Avenue, Suite 203,
>Flushing, NY 11354-1131
>phone 718-321-2873; toll free 800-522-7222
>fax 718-321-3340

Breast Cancer:
National Breast Cancer Coalition
>1707 L Street NW, Suite 1060
>Washington, DC 20036
>phone 202-296-7477
>fax 202-265-6854

Susan G. Komen Breast Cancer Foundation
>National Headquarters
>Occidental Tower, 5005 LBJ Freeway, Suite 370
>Dallas, TX 75244
>phone 214-450-1777; toll free 800-462-9273 or 800-IMAWARE
>fax 214-450-1710

Cancer, General:
American Cancer Society
>1599 Clifton Road NE
>Atlanta, GA 30329-4250
>phone 404-325-3822; toll free 800-227-2345 or 800-ACS-2345

National Cancer Institute of the National Institutes of Health
>phone toll free 800-4-CANCER or 800-422-6237

Cerebral Palsy:
United Cerebral Palsy Association, Inc.
>1660 L Street NW
>Washington, DC 20036-5602
>phone 202-776-0406 or toll free 800-872-5827 or 800-USA-5UCP
>fax 202-776-0414

Charcot-Marie-Tooth Disease:
Charcot-Marie-Tooth Association
> 601 Upland Avenue
> Upland, PA 19015-2494
> phone 610-499-7486; toll free 800-606-2682 or 800-606-CMTA
> fax 610-499-7487

Cystic Fibrosis:
Cystic Fibrosis Foundation
> 6931 Arlington Road
> Bethesda, MD 20814
> phone 301-951-4422; toll free 800-344-4823 or 800-FIGHT-CF

Down Syndrome:
National Association for Down Syndrome
> P. O. Box 4542
> Oak Brook, IL 60522-4542

National Down Syndrome Congress
> 1605 Chantilly Drive, Suite 250
> Atlanta, GA 30324-3269
> phone 404-633-1555; toll free 800-232-6372 or 800-232-NDSC

National Down Syndrome Society
> 666 Broadway, 8th Floor
> New York, NY 10012-2317
> phone 212-460-9330; toll free 800-221-4602
> fax 212-979-2873

Fragile X Syndrome: *(see also Mental Retardation)*
FRAXA Research Foundation, Inc.
> P.O. Box 935
> West Newbury, MA 01985-0935
> phone 978-462-1866
> fax 978-463-9985

Gaucher Disease:

National Gaucher Foundation

      11140 Rockville Pike, Suite 350

      Rockville, MD 20852-3106

      phone 301-816-1515; toll free 800-GAUCHER or 800-925-8885

      fax 301-816-1516

Heart Disease:

American Heart Association

      phone toll free 800-242-8721 or 800-AHA-USA1

Hemophilia:

National Hemophilia Foundation

      116 West 32nd Street, 11th Floor

      New York, NY 10001

      phone 212-328-3700

      fax 212-328-3777

Huntington's Disease:

Huntington's Disease Society of America

      159 West 29th Street, 7th Floor

      New York, NY 10001-5300

      phone 212-242-1968; toll free 800-345-HDSA

Incontinentia Pigmenti:

National Eye Institute

      Building 31, Room 6A32

      Bethesda, MD 20892-2510

      phone 301-496-5248

National Institute of Arthritis and Musculoskeletal and Skin Disorders
> Building 31, Room 4C05
> Bethesda, MD 20892-2350
> phone 301-496-8188

National Organization for Rare Disorders, Inc. (NORD)
> P. O. Box 8923
> New Fairfield, CT 06812-8923
> phone 203-746-6518; toll free 800-999-6673
> fax 203-746-6481

Kidney Disease:
National Kidney Foundation
> 30 East 33rd Street
> New York, NY 10016
> phone toll free 800-622-9010

Liver Disease:
American Liver Foundation
> 1425 Pompton Avenue
> Cedar Grove, NJ 07009
> phone toll free 800-465-4837 or 800-GO-LIVER

Lung Disease:
American Lung Association
> phone toll free 800-LUNG-USA or 800-586-4872

Marfan Syndrome:
National Marfan Foundation
> 382 Main Street
> Port Washington, NY 11050
> phone 516-883-8712; toll free 800-8MARFAN or 800-862-7326
> fax 516-883-8040

Mental Retardation:

American Association on Mental Retardation

444 North Capitol Street NW, Suite 846

Washington, DC 20001-1512

phone 202-387-1968; toll free 800-424-3688

fax 202-387-2193

Mitochondrial Disease:

National Organization for Rare Disorders, Inc. (NORD)

P. O. Box 8923

New Fairfield, CT 06812-8923

phone 203-746-6518; toll free 800-999-6673

fax 203-746-6481

Muscular Dystrophy:

Muscular Dystrophy Association

3300 East Sunrise Drive

Tucson, AZ 85718

phone toll free 800-572-1717

Neurofibromatosis:

National Neurofibromatosis Foundation, Inc.

95 Pine Street, 16th Floor

New York, NY 10005

phone 212-344-6633; toll free 800-323-7938

fax 212-747-0004

Osteogenesis Imperfecta:

Osteogenesis Imperfecta Foundation, Inc.

804 W. Diamond Avenue, Suite 204

Gaithersburg, MD 20878

phone 301-947-0083

fax 301-947-0456

Prader-Willi Syndrome:
Prader-Willi Syndrome Association
>   5700 Midnight Pass Road
>   Sarasota, FL 34242
>   phone 941-312-0400; toll free 800-926-4797
>   fax 941-312-0142

Sickle Cell Disease:
Sickle Cell Disease Association of America
>   200 Corporate Pointe, Suite 495
>   Culver City, CA 90230
>   phone 310-216-6363; toll free 800-421-8453
>   fax 310-215-3722

Tay-Sachs Disease:
National Tay-Sachs and Allied Diseases Association, Inc.
>   2001 Beacon Street, Suite 204
>   Brookline, MA 02146
>   phone 617-277-4463; toll free 800-906-8723
>   fax 617-277-0134

Tuberous Sclerosis:
National Tuberous Sclerosis Association, Inc.
>   8181 Professional Place, Suite 110
>   Landover, MD 20785-2226
>   phone toll free 800-225-6872
>   fax 301-459-0394

Turner Syndrome:
Turner's Syndrome Society of the United States
>   1313 Southeast 5th Street, Suite 327
>   Minneapolis, MN 55414
>   phone toll free 800-365-9944
>   fax 612-379-3619

Urea Cycle Disorders:
National Urea Cycle Disorders Foundation
P.O. Box 32
Sayreville, NJ 08872
phone toll free 800-38N-UCDF or 800-386-8233

Williams Syndrome:
Williams Syndrome Association
P.O. Box 297
Clawson, MI 48017-0297
phone 248-541-3630
fax 248-541-3631

Wilson's Disease:
Wilson's Disease Association
4 Navaho Drive
Brookfield, CT 06810
phone 203-775-4664; toll free 800-399-0266

Xeroderma Pigmentosum:
Xeroderma Pigmentosum Society
P.O. Box 4759
Poughkeepsie, NY 12601

CHAPTER TWENTY-SEVEN

Medical Genetics
on the Internet

More and more health and medical information is becoming available across the Internet, and there are some high quality resources you should know about. Access to physicians, foundations, and support groups is also increasingly available on the Internet.

The following list contains Web site addresses (at press time) for some of the most commonly diagnosed genetic diseases. The site in which you have an interest may not be listed here. Also, new sites appear frequently and some important ones may be available by the time you read this book.

The Web sites listed here were found using two approaches that will be useful if the organization for which you are searching is not here. First, use one of the Internet search engines such as Netscape, Lycos, Yahoo!, or Infoseek. Type in the name of the disease about which you are interested. Run the search and see what comes up. Often you will find access to information and the names of organizations this way. Second, if you already know the name of the group or organization, you can use that as the search term in the Web search. This is a very effective way of finding the Internet home pages of the groups you seek.

If it is information that you are looking for, try Web sites such as the National Institutes of Health, National Library of Medicine, the American Boards of Medical Genetics and Genetic Counseling, the American College of Medical Genetics, the American Society of Human Genetics and Online Mendelian Inheritance in Man, or some of the other general and specific sites listed in this chapter.

If what you are looking for is not listed here, many additional support groups, physicians, and organizations can be found through the Web sites of general groups such as The Alliance of Genetic Support Groups, the March of Dimes, the Council of Regional Networks for Genetic Services, the National Society for Genetic Counselors, and others. Some of these groups act as clearinghouses and provide lists of many different genetic societies, support groups, and research foundations. In addition, some of these groups can provide physician referrals in your area.

If you still cannot find the information you are looking for, try following the advice in Chapter 25 on finding a genetics professional in your area. Contact with such an individual may help you to find the resources you want.

Many of the organizations and support groups for genetic diseases will have listserv/email lists where patients and families can communicate with one another through the Internet to share information, experiences, and emotional or psychological support.

Finally, Web rings are a new way of navigating the Internet. Web rings group interesting sites that focus on a particular subject. This type of grouping facilitates access to the sites by Internet users. As the use of Web rings becomes more popular, many new sites and a greater number of subjects are likely to be included in rings. Web rings have the potential to greatly simplify a search for information on a particular topic. However, unless a Web ring has an extensive resource list, traditional Web searches may also be required to assure access to the greatest number of sources.

The following list is neither an endorsement of any group nor an assurance of the accuracy of any information you might obtain. Remember, almost anyone can put information on the Internet, so always know the source of your information, check the qualifications of the individuals posting the information, and check with your doctor or genetics professional to assure the accuracy of the information you have found and its relevance to your concerns.

General Resources

Alliance of Genetic Support Groups
> http://www.medhelp.org/geneticalliance
> email: info@geneticalliance.org

American Board of Genetic Counseling
> http://www.faseb.org/genetics/abgc/abgcmenu.htm

American Board of Medical Genetics
> http://www.faseb.org/genetics/abmg/abmgmenu.htm

American College of Medical Genetics
> http://www.faseb.org/genetics/acmg/acmgmenu.htm

American Society of Human Genetics
> http://www.faseb.org/genetics/ashg/ashgmenu.htm

Biomednet
> http://biomednet.com

The Council of Regional Networks for Genetic Services (CORN)
> http://www.cc.emory.edu/PEDIATRICS/corn/corn.htm
> (Click on the "contact information" button)

GeneNet: A Worldwide Resource for Genetics
> http://www.genenet.com

Healthgate Data Corp
> http://www.healthgate.com

HealthWorld Online
> http://healthy.net/index.html

Howard Hughes Medical Institute
> http://www.hhmi.org

Human Genome Project
> http://www.ornl.gov/TechResources/Human_Genome/tko/index.htm

March of Dimes Birth Defects Foundation
> http://www.modimes.org

Med Help International

http://www.medhelp.org

Mediconsult

http://www.mediconsult.com

National Center for Biotechnology Information

http://www.ncbi.nlm.nih.gov

National Human Genome Research Institute

http://www.nhgri.nih.gov

National Institutes of Health

http://www.nih.gov/health

National Library of Medicine

http://www.nlm.nih.gov

National Organization for Rare Disorders, Inc. (NORD)

http://www.rarediseases.org

National Society of Genetic Counselors (NSGC)

http://www.nsgc.org

New York Online Access to Health, also called NOAH

This site provides links to the March of Dimes and many
other sites for specific diseases and general health topics.
http://www.noah.cuny.edu

Online Mendelian Inheritance in Man

http://www.ncbi.nlm.nih.gov/Omim

United States Congress: Library of Congress

http://thomas.loc.gov/home/thomas2.html

United Way Help Line

http://www.unitedwaydenver.org/iris/keyw_g.htm
(select Genetic diseases)

Specific Groups and Topics

Achondroplasia

> Little People of America
>
> > http://www.lpaonline.org

Alpha-1 Antitrypsin Deficiency

> Alpha-1 National Association. Alpha-1 antitrypsin deficiency liver disease
>
> > http://www.alpha1.org

Angelman Syndrome

> Angelman Syndrome Foundation, USA
>
> > http://chem-faculty.ucsd.edu/harvey/asfsite

Ataxias

> National Ataxia Foundation
>
> > http://www.ataxia.org

Blood Disorders (see also Hemophilia)

> Cooley Anemia Foundation, Inc.
>
> > http://www.thalassemia.org

Breast Cancer

> National Breast Cancer Coalition
>
> > http://www.natlbcc.org
>
> Susan G. Komen Breast Cancer Foundation
>
> > http://www.mediconsult.com/breast/shareware/komen/bcf.html

Cancer, General

> American Cancer Society
>
> > http://cancer.org/frames.html
>
> National Cancer Institute of the National Institutes of Health
>
> > http://cancernet.nci.nih.gov/icichome.htm
> >
> > http://cancernet.nci.nih.gov/clinpdq/pif.html

Cerebral Palsy

> United Cerebral Palsy Association, Inc.
>
> > http://www.ucpa.org

Charcot-Marie-Tooth Disease

Charcot-Marie-Tooth Association

http://www.charcot-marie-tooth.org

Cystic Fibrosis

Cystic Fibrosis Foundation

http://www.cff.org

Down Syndrome

National Association for Down Syndrome

http://www.nads.org

National Down Syndrome Congress

http://members.carol.net/~ndsc

National Down Syndrome Society

http://www.ndss.org

Fragile X Syndrome (see also Mental Retardation)

FRAXA Research Foundation

http://www.fraxa.org

National Fragile X Foundation

http://www.medhelp.org/www/fragilex

Gaucher Disease

National Gaucher Foundation

http://www.gaucherdisease.org

Heart Disease

American Heart Association

http://www.amhrt.org

http://www.americanheart.org

http://www.americanheart.org/catalog/Scientific_catpage87.html

Hemophilia

National Hemophilia Foundation

http://www.hemophilia.org

Huntington Disease

Huntington's Disease Society of America

http://neuro-www2.mgh.harvard.edu/hdsa/hdsamain.nclk

Incontinentia Pigmenti

> National Organization for Rare Disorders, Inc. (NORD)
>> http://www.rarediseases.org

Kidney Disease

> National Kidney Foundation
>> http://www.kidney.org

Liver Disease

> American Liver Foundation
>> http://gi.ucsf.edu/alf/alffinal/homepagealf.html
>> http://www.liverfoundation.org

Lung Disease

> American Lung Association
>> http://www.lungusa.org

Marfan Syndrome

> National Marfan Foundation
>> http://www.marfan.org

Mental Retardation

> American Association on Mental Retardation
>> http://www.aamr.org

Mitochondrial Disease

> Mitochondrial and Metabolic Disease Center (UCSD)
>> http://biochemgen.ucsd.edu/mmdc/index.htm

Muscular Dystrophy

> Muscular Dystrophy Association
>> http://www.mdausa.org:80

Neurofibromatosis

> National Neurofibromatosis Foundation, Inc.
>> http://www.nf.org

Osteogenesis Imperfecta

> Osteogenesis Imperfecta Foundation, Inc.
>> http://www.oif.org

Prader-Willi Syndrome

    Prader-Willi Syndrome Association

      http://www.pwsausa.org

Sickle Cell Disease

    Sickle Cell Disease Association of America

      http://sicklecelldisease.org

Tay-Sachs Disease

    National Tay Sachs and Allied Disease Association, Inc.

      http://mcrcr2.med.nyu.edu/murphp01/taysachs.htm

Tuberous Sclerosis

    National Tuberous Sclerosis Association, Inc.

      http://www.ntsa.org

Turner Syndrome

    Turner's Syndrome Society of the United States

      http://www.turner-syndrome-us.org

Urea Cycle Disorders

    National Urea Cycle Disorders Foundation

      http://www.NUCDF.org

Williams Syndrome

    Williams Syndrome Association

      http://www.williams-syndrome.org

Wilson's Disease

    Wilson's Disease Association

      http://www.medhelp.org/wda/wil.htm

Xeroderma Pigmentosum

    Xeroderma Pigmentosum Society

      http://www.xps.org

CHAPTER TWENTY-EIGHT

Additional Reading and The Medical Literature

Additional Reading

Biochemistry, 4th ed., 1995. Lubert Stryer. W. H. Freeman and Co. New York

Clinical Genetics Handbook, 2nd ed., 1993. Arthur Robinson, and Mary G. Linden. Blackwell Scientific Publications, Inc., Cambridge, Mass.

Genes V, 1994. Benjamin Lewin. Oxford University Press. Oxford, New York, Tokyo

Genetics, 3rd ed., 1994. David L. Hartl. Jones and Bartlett Publishers, Boston

Genetics and You, 1996. John F. Jackson. Humana Press, Inc. Totowa, N.J.

Human Genetics, 1990. Gordon Edlin. Jones and Bartlett Publishers, Boston

Human Genetics: Problems and Approaches. 3rd ed., 1996. F. Vogel, and A. G. Motulsky. Springer-Verlag. Berlin

Mendelian Inheritance in Man. 11th ed., 1994. Victor A. McKusick. The Johns Hopkins University Press. Baltimore

The Metabolic and Molecular Bases of Inherited Disease, 7th ed., 1995. Charles R. Scriver, Arthur L. Beaudet, William S. Sly, and David Valle, editors. McGraw-Hill, Inc. New York

Molecular Biology of the Cell, 3rd ed., 1994. Bruce Alberts, Dennis Bray, Julian Lewis, Martin Raff, Keith Roberts, and James D. Watson. Garland Publishing, Inc. New York, London

Principles of Medical Genetics, 1990. Thomas D. Gelehrter, and Francis S. Collins. Williams and Wilkins. Baltimore

Signs of Life: The Language and Meanings of DNA, 1995. Robert Pollack. Houghton Mifflin. Boston

Thompson and Thompson: Genetics in Medicine, 5th ed., 1991. Margaret
W. Thompson, Roderick R. McInnes, and Huntington F. Willard.
W. B. Saunders and Co., Harcourt Brace Jovanovich, Inc.
Philadelphia

Children's Books

Amazing Schemes within Your Genes, 1993. Dr. Fran Balkwill. Carolrhoda
Books, Inc. Minneapolis
Cells Are Us, 1993. Dr. Fran Balkwill. Carolrhoda Books, Inc. Minneapolis.
DNA Is Here To Stay, 1993. Dr. Fran Balkwill. Carolrhoda Books, Inc.
Minneapolis
The Cell Works Microexplorers, 1997. Patrick A. Baeverle, and Norbert
Landa. Barron's Educational Series, Inc. Hauppauge, N.Y.
Ingenious Genes, 1997. Patrick A. Baeverle, and Norbert Landa. Barron's
Educational Series, Inc. Hauppauge, N.Y.
How the Y Makes the Guy Microexplorers, 1997. Patrick A. Baeverle, and
Norbert Landa. Barron's Educational Series, Inc. Hauppauge, N.Y.
Double Talking Helix Blues, 1993. Joel Herskowitz, Ira Herskowitz, and
Judy Cuddihy. Cold Spring Harbor Press, N.Y.

Using the Medical Literature

For many specific topics in genetics, there is information available in
brochure form. Printed literature about specific diseases, tests, or treatment
options may be available through your physician or genetics professional.
In addition, your local bookseller may carry or be able to get books on specific topics in genetics or medicine. Some cities have bookstores that spe-
cialize in scientific or medical books. A number of booksellers are also
accessible via the Internet.

Your local library may be another good source for books on specific topics in genetics. Ask the librarian for help if you are not familiar with how to
locate and use the available resources.

Finally, you may want to try to access scientific literature databases such as Medline or Cancerlit. These databases contain references for primary scientific research and review articles, much of which is written and intended for the scientific community, not the general public. Some of the scientific data and results may be difficult to interpret accurately for those who do not have a background in science or medicine. Individuals should always consult with their physicians regarding the information they find and the accuracy of their interpretations.

The literature database called Medline contains references for basic science research and review articles. Medline can be accessed online through a variety of resources:

- Biomednet
  http://biomednet.com
- HealthGate Data Corp
  http://www.healthgate.com
- HealthWorld Online
  http://healthy.net/index.html
- The National Center for Biotechnology Information
  http://www.ncbi.nlm.nih.gov
- The National Library of Medicine
  http://www.nlm.nih.gov

The literature database called Cancerlit contains references for basic science research and review articles with special attention to articles on cancer. Cancerlit can also be accessed online:

- HealthGate Data Corp.
  http://www.healthgate.com
- The National Library of Medicine
  http://www.nlm.nih.gov
  http://www.nlm.nih.gov/databases/databases.html

Keeping Up with Genetics News

Many sources can help you keep up with new developments in genetic research. These include television and newspapers as well as Internet sources such as those for the Human Genome Project, the National Institutes of Health, the American Cancer Society, The March of Dimes, and many other general resources listed here and in previous chapters.

As you find Web sites, support groups, and physician resources that meet your needs and interests, you will also identify the news sources that work best for you. Many groups publish newsletters or post new information on the Internet regularly. Remember, select with care only reliable sources of your information and check any new information with your geneticist to verify its accuracy and relevance to your medical concerns.

Epilogue

Genetic science promises to make great changes in the management of patients and families with many different kinds of medical problems. We are only beginning to see the impact that genetic research and testing will have on all of our lives and on the practice of medicine in the new century. As additional genes are discovered and the genetic influences on our health are characterized, the number of conditions that can be individually assessed will continue to expand. As the causes of genetic diseases become better understood, new preventions, treatments, and cures for diseases of all kinds are likely to become common practice.

For the promise of genetics to be fulfilled, it is vital that private and federal support of genetic research continue. It is vital that gene discoveries and new knowledge be made available for widespread utilization by doctors and patients without impediment or unnecessary restriction from patents or ownership rights. It is also vital that the public understand the applications and benefits of genetic research.

Education about genetics is necessary so that people can make informed health-care decisions for themselves and their families. As people better understand the principles and concepts of genetics and health, they will be better equipped to make decisions about genetic testing and treatment options. Understanding also protects people from false expectations, unrealistic hopes, and sensationalized or exaggerated claims about the significance of specific breakthroughs in genetics.

Individuals concerned with inheritance or transmission of genetic diseases should be aware of the options for medical care and support in genetics. We as a society must maintain a health-care system that allows individuals the opportunity to seek the medical support they feel is important, to obtain the latest information and treatments, and to participate in the medical decisions that affect their lives.

Appendix

Guide to Genetic Diseases

There are thousands of human traits, conditions, or diseases that are known or suspected to be genetically influenced. What follows is clearly a very abbreviated list. Further information on these and many other traits, conditions, and diseases can be found in the resources listed in Chapters 25 through 28 and the Bibliography.

Disease/Trait	Pattern of Inheritance/ Genetic Alteration	Incidence[1]	Comments
Achondroplasia	sporadic, AD[2]	1 in 20,000	87.5 % of cases are new mutations
Adrenoleukodystrophy (ALD)	2 forms; XL, AR	1 in 100,000	female carriers of XL ALD can show moderate to severe symptoms; neonatal ALD is AR
Alpha-1 antitrypsin deficiency	AR	variable; 1 in 2,500 Caucasians	important contributor to lung and liver disease; aggravated by smoking and other environmental agents; carriers may be at increased risk for lung disease
Alport syndrome	AR, XLR forms; possible AD form	unknown	syndrome of deafness with kidney disease
Alzheimer's disease	sporadic, AD, MF; possible MITO form	1 in 50 in United States	at least 50 % of cases sporadic
Amyotrophic lateral sclerosis (ALS, Lou Gehrig's disease)	sporadic, AD	1 in 70,000	10 % of cases familial; 3 familial forms
Anencephaly (see neural tube defects)			
Angelman syndrome (AS)	most cases sporadic	NF[3]	shows imprinting effect; commonly caused by deletion of chromosome 15q11-q13; some cases due to AD single gene or AD imprinting mutation
Apert syndrome	most cases sporadic; AD rare	1 in 160,000	paternal age effect
Biotinidase deficiency	AR	1 in 100,000	treated with biotin
Breast cancer	most cases sporadic;10 % familial	overall lifetime risk may be as high as 1 in 10 for women in United States	familial cases AD; shows locus and allelic heterogeneity
Canavan disease	AR	1 in 14,000 Ashkenazi Jewish	less common in other populations
Charcot-Marie-Tooth disease (CMT)	AD, AR, XL, sporadic forms	combined; 1 in 2,500	CMT1A frequently caused by a gene duplication
Cleft Lip/Palate	AD, AR, XL, CHR, MF forms	variable; 1-2 in 1,000	may be an isolated trait or syndromic; complex genetic and environmental factors contribute to many cases
Cockayne syndrome	AR	rare	3 forms; extreme sensitivity to sunlight, ultraviolet radiation

Disease/Trait	Pattern of Inheritance/ Genetic Alteration	Incidence[1]	Comments
Color blindness	classic red-green form is XLR	8 in 100 males of European descent	gene is common; less than 1 % of females are color blind
Colorectal cancer	most cases sporadic; some AD	1 in 20	shows locus and allelic heterogeneity
Congenital adrenal hyperplasia	several forms; all AR	variable; 1 in 10,000-25,000 in Europe and North America	21-hydroxylase deficiency is most common form; salt-losing form can cause lethal electrolyte imbalance in neonates
Congenital heart defects	5-6 % CHR; 3-5 % AD, AR, XL; 85-90 % MF	0.8 in 100	may be an isolated trait or syndromic
Coronary artery disease	many forms; AR, AD, XL, MF	1 in 15 in some Western populations	genetic and nongenetic risk factors exist
Cri-du-chat syndrome	sporadic	1 in 50,000	most cases caused by deletion of chromosome 5p; some cases caused by inheritance of a parental translocation
Cystic fibrosis	AR	1 in 2,500 Caucasians	1 in 3,300 Ashkenazi Jewish
Deafness	AR, AD, XL, MITO, MF, nongenetic forms	1 in 1,000 newborns; prevalence increases with age	may be an isolated trait or syndromic; extreme locus and allelic heterogeneity
Diabetes mellitus:			
Type I Insulin dependent diabetes (IDDM)	MF	1 in 200	autoimmune disease
Type II Noninsulin dependent diabetes (NIDDM)	several forms; AD, MF	1 in 20 worldwide	genetically heterogeneous
Maturity onset diabetes (MODY)	3 forms; all AD		NIDDM subtype; 3 different genes identified
DiGeorge syndrome	sporadic, AD	1 in 4,000	commonly caused by deletion of chromosome 22q11.2; significant overlap with Velocardiofacial syndrome (VCFS, see VCFS)
Down syndrome	sporadic/CHR	overall, 1 in 600	also known as Trisomy 21; maternal age effect
Duchenne muscular dystrophy	sporadic, XLR	1 in 3,000 males	30 % of cases are new mutations

Disease/Trait	Pattern of Inheritance/ Genetic Alteration	Incidence[1]	Comments
Epidermolysis bullosa	many forms; most AD, also AR	1 in 50,000	can range in severity from mild to lethal; shows genetic heterogeneity
Epilepsy	complex; MF, nongenetic forms	1 in 100	may be isolated trait or syndromic; clear genetic causes comprise a relatively small percentage of cases
Fabry disease	XLR	1 in 40,000	carrier females may show mild symptoms
Familial adenomatous polyposis (FAP)	AD	variable; 1 in 13,000 in Danish populations	predisposition to colon cancer
Familial hypercholesterolemia	AD	very frequent; 1 in 500	elevated serum cholesterol; predisposition to coronary artery disease
Fanconi anemia	several forms; all AR	variable	shows locus and allelic heterogeneity
Fragile X syndrome	XL	1 in 1,250 males; 1 in 2,000 females	caused by expansion of a trinucleotide repeat; 30-50 % of female carriers show signs of mental retardation; shows anticipation
Friedreich's ataxia	AR	1 in 50,000	majority of cases caused by expansion of a trinucleotide repeat; does not show anticipation
Galactosemia	AR	1 in 60,000	neonatal testing common; treated by dietary restriction of galactose
Gaucher disease	AR	variable; 1 in 900 Ashkenazi Jewish births	3 types, each with different clinical course
Glucose 6-phosphate dehydrogenase deficiency (G6PD)	XLR	variable; as high as 1 in 5 males in some parts of Africa	most common enzyme deficiency in humans; most affected individuals show symptoms only with certain medications, infections or ingestion of fava beans
Hemophilia A	XLR	1 in 10,000 male births	also known as Factor VIII deficiency; historical note, European royal families from Queen Victoria to Russia were affected by either Hemophilia A or B

Disease/Trait	Pattern of Inheritance/ Genetic Alteration	Incidence[1]	Comments
Hemophilia B	XLR	1 in 30,000 males	also known as Factor IX deficiency or Christmas disease
Hereditary fructose intolerance (HFI)	AR	unclear; 1 in 20,000 in Swiss populations	patients develop a strong distaste for fructose or sucrose containing foods
Hereditary hemochromatosis	AR	common, 1 in 330	if untreated, complications can include diabetes, liver damage and heart failure
Hereditary neuropathy with liability to pressure palsies (HNPP)	sporadic, AD	unknown	gene deletion on chromosome 17p; deletion of same gene that is duplicated in CMT1A
Hereditary nonpolyposis colon cancer (HNPCC)	AD	unclear	at least 5 different genes involved; contribution of mutation in these genes to many sporadic colon cancers is probable
Homocystinuria	AR	variable; 1 in 200,000	pharmacologic use of folic acid helpful; risk factor for coronary artery disease
Hunter syndrome	XLR	less than 1 in 20,000	symptoms can vary from severe to mild
Huntington disease	AD	variable; 1 in 14,000 in Western European populations; higher in others	caused by expansion of a trinucleotide repeat; shows anticipation
Hurler syndrome	AR	less than 1 in 20,000	allelic with Scheie and Hurler-Scheie syndromes
Hypertension	MF, genetic and environmental risk factors exist	1 in 5	may be an isolated trait or syndromic
Incontinentia pigmenti	XLD	unclear	affected males not seen; thought to be lethal in male fetuses
Kennedy's disease	XLR	1 in 50,000 males	also called spinobulbar muscular atrophy; caused by expansion of a trinucleotide repeat in the androgen receptor gene
Klinefelter syndrome	sporadic/CHR	1 in 1,000 male live births	affected individuals carry 47 chromosomes- 2 X chromosomes in the presence of 1 Y; common cause of hypogonadism in males

Disease/Trait	Pattern of Inheritance/ Genetic Alteration	Incidence[1]	Comments
Leber's hereditary optic neuropathy (LHON)	MITO	NF	variable disease course
Lesch-Nyhan syndrome (LN)	sporadic, XLR	rare	hyperuricemia, mental retardation and self-mutilatory behavior
Lipoprotein lipase deficiency	AR	1 in 1,000,000	elevated triglyceride levels characteristic; no apparent predisposition to atherosclerosis
Lowe syndrome	XLR	NF	most female carriers can be detected by eye exam
Maple syrup urine disease (MSUD)	AR	1 in 185,000	treated by dietary restriction of branched chain amino acids; neonatal testing common
Marfan syndrome	sporadic, AD	1 in 10,000	15-30 % of cases are new mutations; highly variable disease expression
McArdle disease	AR	NF	also known as Glycogen storage disease type V; adult and rare infantile forms
Menkes disease	XLR	1 in 50,000-100,000	sparse hair, neurodegenerative disease; defect in copper transport
Mucopolysaccharidosis	several types; all AR except Hunter (XLR)		see Hunter, Hurler, Sanfilippo syndromes
Multiple endocrine neoplasia (MEN)	2 types; both AD	1 in 20,000 combined	predisposition to particular cancers; shows locus and allelic heterogeneity
Multiple sclerosis (MS)	MF	1 in 1,000	autoimmune disease
Myoclonic epilepsy, lactic acidosis, and stroke like episodes (MELAS)	MITO	NF	defect in mitochondrial translation or RNA processing
Myoclonic epilepsy with ragged red fibers (MERRF)	MITO	NF	defect in mitochondrial translation of RNA processing
Myotonic dystrophy (DM)	AD	1 in 8,000	caused by expansion of a trinucleotide repeat; shows anticipation

230

Disease/Trait	Pattern of Inheritance/ Genetic Alteration	Incidence[1]	Comments
Nephrogenic diabetes insipidus	2 simple genetic types; AD, XL	NF	nongenetic, acquired disease can occur in reaction to certain drugs; may also be syndromic
Neural tube defects	MF, syndromic forms	1 in 1,000 in United States	supplementation of mother's diet with folic acid helpful; 0.4 mg daily folic acid supplement recommended for all women of child bearing age
Neurofibromatosis Type 1 (NF1), von Recklinghausen's disease	sporadic, AD	1 in 3,000	Neurofibromatosis Type 2 also sporadic, AD; 1 in 40,000
Niemann Pick disease	several forms; all AR	type A, 1 in 40,000 Ashkenazi Jewish; type B, 1 in 80,000 Ashkenazi Jewish	types A and B are allelic (caused by mutations in the same gene)
Osteogenesis imperfecta (OI)	several inherited forms, most AD, AR less common; also sporadic	1 in 5,000-10,000	different types can vary from mild to progressive to lethal
Otosclerosis	apparent AD with reduced penetrance	1 in 100, possibly higher	gene recently mapped
Phenylketonuria (PKU)	AR	variable; 1 in 12,000 Caucasians, 1 in 16,000 Asians	treated by dietary restriction of phenylalanine; neonatal testing common
Polycystic kidney disease (PKD)	AD, AR forms	adult ADPKD may be as high as 1 in 400-1,000	may be an isolated trait or syndromic; up to 11 % of end stage renal disease may be genetic
Pompe disease	AR	1 in 50,000-100,000	also known as Glycogen storage disease type II; infantile, juvenile and adult forms
Porphyria	AD, AR forms	variable; most common form 1 in 10,000	disruption of heme biosynthesis
Prader-Willi syndrome (PWS)	most cases sporadic	1 in 20,000	most cases due to deletion of chromosome 15q11.2-q12; some cases due to imprinting defect
Refsum disease	AR	rare	treated by dietary restriction of phytanic acid
Retinitis pigmentosa (RP)	AR, AD, XLR forms	1 in 4,000 combined	important cause of progressive vision loss

Disease/Trait	Pattern of Inheritance/ Genetic Alteration	Incidence[1]	Comments
Retinoblastoma	majority sporadic; also AD	1 in 18,000	high penetrance; deletions of chromosome 13q14 common
Sanfilippo syndrome	AR	less than 1 in 20,000	4 types; most common mucopolysaccharidosis (see Hunter, Hurler, Mucopolysaccharidosis)
Sickle cell anemia	AR	1 in 625 African Americans	variable disease course
Smith-Magenis syndrome	sporadic/CHR	1 in 25,000	deletion of chromosome 17p11.2
Spina bifida (see neural tube defects)			
Spinal cerebellar ataxia (SCA)	AD	1 in 20,000	several types; caused by expansion of a trinucleotide repeat; shows anticipation and locus heterogeneity
Spinal muscular atrophy (SMA)	AR	1 in 13,000	3 types classified by severity and age at onset; Type I Werdnig-Hoffman disease most severe
Tay-Sach's disease	AR	1 in 4,000 Ashkenazi Jewish	less common in other populations
Thalassemia:			
Alpha thalassemia	autosomal, complex	most common in individuals of Mediterranean and Asian descent	commonly caused by deletions of alpha globin genes; humans carry 2 alpha globin genes on each chromosome 16; deletion of 4 genes results in hydrops fetalis (alpha thalassemia), deletion of 3 gene results in chronic hemolytic anemia (Hemoglobin H disease), deletion of 2 genes results in mild anemia (alpha thalassemia trait), deletion of 1 gene is a silent carrier state
Beta thalassemia major	AR	variable; 1 in 400-20,000	severe anemia
Beta thalassemia minor	beta thalassemia carrier state	variable; average, 3 in 100 worldwide	can result in mild anemia
Trisomy 13	sporadic/CHR	1 in 15,000	maternal age effect
Trisomy 18	sporadic/CHR	1 in 5,000	maternal age effect; 95 % of fetuses spontaneously abort

Disease/Trait	Pattern of Inheritance/ Genetic Alteration	Incidence[1]	Comments
Trisomy 21 (see Down syndrome)			
Tuberous sclerosis	sporadic, AD	1 in 10,000-30,000	60 % of cases are new mutations; shows locus and allelic heterogeneity
Turner syndrome	sporadic/CHR	1 in 1,500 females	99 % of fetuses spontaneously abort
Velocardiofacial syndrome (VCFS)	sporadic, AD	unclear	large overlap with DiGeorge syndrome (see DiGeorge)
von Gierke disease	AR	NF	also known as Glycogen storage disease type Ia; treated with a combination of dietary and other therapies
von Willibrand disease	most AD; less common AR	1 in 8,000	several clinical types; may resemble mild Hemophilia A; most common inherited bleeding disorder in humans
Waardenburg syndrome	sporadic, AD	Type 1, 1 in 40,000	3 types; shows locus and allelic heterogeneity
Williams syndrome	sporadic, possible AD form	1 in 10,000	caused by deletion of/in elastin gene on chromosome 7q11.2
Wilms tumor	sporadic, AD	1 in 10,000	less than 1 % familial AD; deletion of chromosome 11p13 common
Wilson disease	AR	1 in 30,000-40,000	defect in copper metabolism; treated with penacillamine
Xeroderma pigmentosa	AR	1 in 250,000	several forms; caused by DNA repair defect; extreme sensitivity to sunlight; predisposition to cancer
Zellweger syndrome	several forms; all AR	1 in 100,000	shows locus and allelic heterogeneity

[1] Estimates of disease incidence are approximate and can vary among literature sources. The incidence of some genetic disorders and traits can also vary greatly among different ancestral populations.

[2] AD= autosomal dominant; AR= autosomal recessive; XL= X-linked; XLD= X-linked dominant; XLR= X-linked recessive; CHR= chromosomal; MF= multifactorial; MITO= mitochondrial

[3] NF= not found

Glossary

Adenine. Adenine is one of the four nucleotides found in DNA. The nucleotide adenine is also found in RNA. Adenine base pairs across the rungs of the DNA ladder with the nucleotide thymine. In RNA, adenine pairs with uridine. *See "thymine," "uridine."*

Allele. The term allele is used to describe one of the members of a gene pair or, alternatively, one of the different, polymorphic sequences that may exist within a population for a particular gene or segment of DNA.

Amino acid. The amino acid is the basic building block of proteins. Amino acids are found in the cytoplasm of the cells where they are assembled on ribosomes, end-to-end in a string. A string of amino acids makes a protein. There are twenty different amino acids in cells and the same amino acid can be represented by several different RNA codons. *See "codon."*

Amniocentesis. Amniocentesis is a prenatal procedure performed for the purpose of collecting amniotic fluid from the amniotic sac, which surrounds the fetus. The amniotic fluid contains fetal cells that can be used for prenatal diagnosis using genetic testing procedures. Amniotic fluid and cells can also be used for biochemical tests. Amniocentesis is performed by aspiration of amniotic fluid from within the amniotic sac using a needle inserted into the sac through the abdomen. Amniocentesis is usually performed at 16 to 18 weeks of pregnancy and, while generally uncomplicated, can carry certain risks for the fetus including a very low (usually less than 1 percent) risk for miscarriage.

Aneuploid. Aneuploid is a term used to describe cells that do not contain the usual number of chromosomes, forty-six chromosomes in twenty-three pairs. Aneuploid cells can contain extra chromosomes or be missing chromosomes. Some examples of aneuploidy include Down syndrome, which involves the presence of extra chromosome 21 material, and Turner syndrome, which involves the absence of X chromosome material.

Autosome. An autosome is any one of chromosomes 1 through 22. Autosome chromosomes do not include the X and Y chromosomes, which are known as the sex chromosomes.

Base substitution. *See "mutation."*

Cell. A cell is a microscopic, self-contained unit that is the basic building block of tissues, organs, and bodies. A cell is a fluid- and protein-filled entity bound by a membrane that encloses the contents of the cell. The cell membrane is made up of chemical components called phospholipids, which serve to separate the cellular components from the outside environment. Cells, through their genetic information and the synthesis of certain proteins, perform specific metabolic and structural tasks within tissues, organs, and bodies.

Chorionic villus sampling. Chorionic villus sampling, or CVS, is a prenatal procedure performed for the collection of fetal cells from the tissues that surround the fetus. Chorionic villus tissue can be used for prenatal diagnosis using genetic testing or biochemical analyses. CVS is performed by aspiration of chorionic villus tissues from around the fetus using a needle inserted either through the abdomen wall or through the cervix. CVS is usually performed at nine to twelve weeks of pregnancy and, while generally uncomplicated, can carry certain risks for the fetus including a low risk for miscarriage.

Chromosome. A chromosome is the structural component of the genetic material. Chromosomes reside within a part of the cell called the nucleus. Chromosomes are long molecules of DNA that carry genes. There are usually forty-six chromosomes within human cells and these forty-six chromosomes make up twenty-three pairs of like chromosomes.

Chromosomes are passed from generation to generation as the transporters of genes. Chromosomes also contain structural sequences that enable their duplication and assortment during cell division.

Cloning. Cloning is a general term used to describe a variety of genetic methods. The term cloning can be used to describe the isolation and reproduction of an individual gene or group of genes, the isolation and growth of a genetically identical population of cells, the disaggregation of animal embryos to create twinning, or the use of somatic cell nuclear transfer to create an animal genetically identical to the animal from which the nucleus came. *See "somatic cell nuclear transfer."*

Codon. A codon is a grouped sequence of three nucleotides in RNA that specifies a single amino acid. Codons are the basic unit of the genetic code. Codons are used by ribosomes during translation to specify the sequence of amino acids incorporated into the newly forming protein. Because of the four different nucleotides in RNA, there are sixty-four different possible codons but only twenty different amino acids. As a result, the genetic code is said to be redundant—that is, several different codons signal for the same amino acid. Because of this redundancy, some mutations in DNA do not alter the amino acid sequence of the protein because they change the codon to another one that specifies the same amino acid. *See "genetic code."*

Cordocentesis. Cordocentesis, or fetal blood sampling (FBS), is a prenatal procedure performed for the collection of fetal blood directly from the umbilical cord. The blood and cells obtained can be used for prenatal diagnosis using genetic tests or biochemical analyses. Cordocentesis is performed using a needle inserted through the abdominal wall of the mother and into the umbilical cord. Cordocentesis is usually performed after twenty weeks of pregnancy and, while generally uncomplicated, can carry certain risks for the fetus including a low risk for miscarriage.

Cytosine. Cytosine is one of the four nucleotides found in DNA. The nucleotide cytosine is also found in RNA. Cytosine base pairs across the rungs of the DNA ladder with the nucleotide guanine. *See "guanine."*

Deletion mutation. A deletion mutation is a mutation in which genetic material that is supposed to be present is lost. Deletions can be large or small and the consequences of the mutation are often affected by the size and location of the deletion.

Diploid. Diploid is a term used to describe cells that contain the complete content of the human genome, that is forty-six chromosomes in twenty-three pairs. Somatic cells are normally diploid.

DNA. DNA stands for **d**eoxyribo**n**ucleic **a**cid. DNA is the molecule that carries the genetic information used by a cell for the manufacture of proteins. A chromosome is a long molecule of DNA. DNA is made up of individual units called nucleotides that, when joined end to end, form one side of the ladder-like structure of the DNA molecule. The two sides of the ladder pair through hydrogen bonds to complete the two-sided, or double-stranded DNA molecule.

Dominant. The term dominant is often used when describing the physical effect of gene mutations or patterns of inheritance. Dominant mutations are gene mutations that exert a physical effect on the carrier regardless of the concurrent presence of a normal gene.

Dominant negative mutation. Dominant negative mutations are mutations that interrupt a protein in such a way that it interferes with the functioning of the normal protein made by the other allele of a gene pair. For example, if the proteins made by both genes of a gene pair interact to form a structure or perform a function as a multi-unit protein complex, the altered protein may destroy the function of the entire complex. Dominant negative gene mutations can produce more serious effects than would result if the protein were missing entirely, because of the interference caused by the altered protein.

Duplication mutation. A duplication mutation is a mutation in which a segment of genetic material appears more times in the mutation than it would in normal circumstances. Duplication mutations can be large or small. The consequences of the mutation are often affected by the location and size of the duplication.

Egg. The egg is the germ cell produced by the female reproductive system for the formation of an embryo. The egg contains one of each of the twenty-three chromosomes and many other cellular components, including mitochondria. At conception, the egg is fertilized by the sperm from the male.

Enzyme. An enzyme is a protein that catalyzes a biochemical reaction. Some enzymes are made up of single-protein amino acid chains called polypeptides. Other enzymes function as multimers of two or more polypeptides joined together in a complex. Enzyme deficiencies can cause genetic disease either because of the loss of necessary products of enzymatic reactions or because of the buildup of toxic or harmful components of enzymatic reactions.

Exons. An exon is a part of a gene that is retained throughout the modifications that occur after transcription. Exons are used in translation to encode the sequence of a protein. Exons are distinguished from introns, the intervening sequences removed from RNAs before translation. *See "introns."*

Fertilization. Fertilization is the process through which sperm and egg combine. During fertilization, the sperm and egg each contribute one chromosome to each of the twenty-three chromosome pairs.

Fetal blood sampling. *See "cordocentesis."*

Gain of function mutation. A gain of function mutation is a mutation that causes the altered protein to function in a way in which it could not function before the mutation. If this new function is harmful to cells, genetic disease can be the result.

Gene. A gene is the unit of information used by the cell as a blueprint for the manufacture of a protein. Mutations in genes can result in alterations in proteins. Failure of proteins to function properly can result in genetic disease. Genes are carried on chromosomes and are inherited from one generation to the next as chromosomes are passed from parent to child.

Genetic code. The genetic code is the means by which the cell converts the information in DNA and RNA into the function of proteins. First, DNA is transcribed in the nucleus into RNA, then the RNA is transported to the cytoplasm where it is translated by ribosomes. The ribosomes convert the RNA information into amino acids. In the RNA, three nucleotides together in a row specify a single amino acid, and the different possible three-nucleotide sequences are how the ribosome incorporates different amino acids specifically into a protein. With four nucleotides in RNA and three nucleotides in a codon, there are $4 \times 4 \times 4 = 64$ possible different codons. However, there are only twenty different amino acids. As such, several different codons can specify the same amino acid. Because of this feature, the genetic code is said to be redundant. Since the genetic code is redundant, mutations that alter a codon but not the amino acid it represents will not alter the sequence of a protein. Mutations that alter a codon so that it specifies a different amino acid will result in production of an altered protein.

Genome. The genome is the entire complement of the genetic material of an organism. The diploid human genome consists of twenty-three pairs of chromosomes containing an estimated six billion base pairs of DNA and 50,000 to 100,000 different genes. The Human Genome Project is an international research project aimed at determining the sequence of the entire human genome and identifying all of the genes contained therein.

Germ cell. A germ cell is a cell destined to become a sperm or an egg. Sperm and eggs contain one each of the twenty-three different chromosomes. The sperm and eggs from the parents combine at fertilization to reconstitute the genome of forty-six chromosomes.

Gonadal mosaicism. Gonadal mosaicism is a term used to describe the situation when some but not all of the sperm or egg cell precursors in an individual carry a particular DNA sequence. Gonadal mosaicism can occur when a mutation is not inherited from a parent but instead appears during development. Because of the new mutation, some of the individual's cells will carry the mutation and others will not. In gonadal mosaicism there is a risk for passing the mutation to children. The importance of gonadal mosaicism is an increased risk for additional affected children because of the presence of residual sperm or egg precursors that could pass the mutation to a subsequent child.

Guanine. Guanine is one of the four nucleotides found in DNA. The nucleotide guanine is also found in RNA. Guanine base pairs across the rungs of the DNA ladder with the nucleotide cytosine. *See "cytosine."*

Haploid. Haploid is the term used to describe cells that contain only one each of the twenty-three different chromosomes. The chromosomes in haploid cells do not exist as pairs. Sperm and egg cells are haploid.

Independent assortment. Independent assortment is a term used to describe the manner in which chromosomes are sorted to daughter cells during the first cell division of meiosis. Unlike mitosis where one copy of each of the forty-six chromosomes goes to each daughter cell, during the first division of meiosis, the **pairs** of chromosomes are separated such that one chromosome of each pair goes to each of the daughter cells. As a result, the two cells at this stage contain twenty-three chromosomes that are double, or duplicated, chromosomes. Which chromosome of the pair goes to each daughter cell is randomly determined for each of the twenty-three pairs of chromosomes. As such, the sperm and egg do not inherit a complete grand-parental set. Instead, any given sperm or egg will either contain a grand-maternal or grand-paternal chromosome for each of the twenty-three chromosomes in the cell. This results in a shuffling of chromosomes from generation to generation and provides a greater diversity in the sets of genes inherited together.

Insertion mutation. An insertion mutation is a mutation in which genetic material that is not normally present in a region of the genetic material is inserted into the sequence. Insertion mutations can be large or small. The consequences of the mutation are often affected by the size and location of the insertion.

Intervening sequences. The term intervening sequence is often used to describe an intron. Introns are found within the genes of all higher organisms, including plants, animals, and humans. Introns are removed from RNAs before translation (*see "introns"*). The term intervening sequence may also sometimes be used to describe the DNA sequences that span the distance between genes.

Introns. An intron is the portion of a gene that is removed after transcription but before translation. Mutations in introns that disrupt their removal from RNAs can result in the production of altered proteins. The purpose of introns is not clearly understood, but they appear in the genes of all higher organisms. *See "intervening sequences."*

Karyotype. A karyotype is a tool used by cytogeneticists to study the chromosomal content of cells. For karyotype analysis, dividing cells are captured just prior to mitosis and the chromosomes are fixed to a microscope slide. The chromosomes are stained with a dye to generate an alternating pattern of light and dark bands. The bands provide detailed landmarks for analysis of chromosome content. Karyotyping can be performed on many types of cells including amniocytes, CVS tissues, and lymphocytes. Karyotype analysis is capable of identifying alterations in chromosomes such as aneuploidies, deletion mutations, duplication mutations, insertion mutations, rearrangements, and translocations. Karyotype analysis can be performed prenatally or postnatally and is often used in the diagnosis of genetic disease.

Loss of function mutation. A loss of function mutation is one in which a protein is altered so that it can no longer perform the function for which it was originally designed. Loss of function mutations can profoundly influence the function of a cell if they occur in critical proteins.

Meiosis. Meiosis is the process of cell division that occurs in germ cells whereby cellular DNA is duplicated, followed by two consecutive cell divisions. During meiosis, sperm and eggs reduce their chromosome number from forty-six to twenty-three to preserve the amount of the genetic material from generation to generation. In the first division of meiosis the pairs of like chromosomes are separated such that each daughter cell receives a single chromosome of each pair. At this stage, each of the two daughter cells contains twenty-three double or duplicated chromosomes. In the second cell division, this duplicated chromosome is divided so that each daughter cell receives twenty-three single chromosomes. *See "independent assortment" and "recombination."*

Mitochondria. Mitochondria are the power plants of cells. They are responsible for producing the energy that cells use to perform tasks. Mitochondria carry circular DNA molecules that encode a dozen or so proteins. Mitochondria also contain other components such as RNA and proteins. Each cell contains many mitochondria. During cell division, mitochondria are assorted to the daughter cells. Mitochondria and their DNA are inherited through eggs and not through sperm. Mutations in mitochondrial DNA are passed from mothers to children and not from fathers. The severity of mitochondrial mutations depends upon many factors, including the number of mutant mito-chondria contained in a cell and the precise mutation present.

Mitosis. Mitosis is the process whereby cells duplicate each of their forty-six chromosomes and then split into two cells, dividing the genetic material so that each daughter cell receives one each of the forty-six chromosomes. The function of mitosis is to produce new cells. Mitosis occurs throughout the body and throughout growth and development to produce the billions of cells that make up the organs and tissues of the body.

Mutagens. Mutagens are substances that can cause mutations in DNA. Mutagens include chemicals and other substances such as radiation and ultraviolet (UV) light. The effects of mutagens on the body generally depend upon the time of exposure, the location of the exposure, and the dose of the mutagen. Exposure to large amounts of mutagen early in development is potentially very damaging to the individual because a large percentage of cells could be damaged. Mutagens have also been found to be able to cause cancer by damaging DNA in genes critical for control of cell growth.

Mutation. A mutation is a change in the sequence of a piece of DNA. Some mutations can be deleterious to the function of proteins, resulting in disease, while other mutations may not be harmful. Mutations that are not harmful to the functioning of a protein are sometimes called polymorphisms or base substitutions instead of mutations to denote their lack of harmful effect. Mutations can be deletions, duplications, insertions, inversions, rearrangements, or point mutations.

Nucleotide. The nucleotide is the basic chemical component of DNA and RNA. Nucleotides are the chemical alphabet of biology. Many nucleotides strung together make up the sequence of the DNA and RNA. There are four basic nucleotides in DNA that, when combined in different combinations, specify the sequence of the encoded proteins. All organisms use the same four nucleotides in DNA. The nucleotides in DNA are adenine, cytosine, guanine, and thymine. RNA does not use thymine but instead uses the nucleotide uridine in its place. In DNA, nucleotides base pair across the rungs of the molecular ladder to form a double-stranded DNA molecule that is very stable. RNA is not double stranded. The precise base pairing feature of nucleotides is used by the cell in the duplication of the DNA and in the production of RNA, and by scientists interested in studying DNA sequences. *See "adenine," "cytosine," "guanine," "thymine," and "uridine."*

Nucleus. The nucleus is the compartment of the cell that contains the DNA. The nucleus is separated from the other regions of the cell by the nuclear membrane, which helps to contain the DNA and other nuclear components. The nucleus exists within the confines of the cell membrane and is the location of transcription. The nuclear membrane breaks down during mitosis to facilitate the separation of the chromosomes into the newly forming daughter cells and then subsequently reforms after cell division is complete.

Point mutation. A point mutation is a single base change that occurs within a sequence of DNA. Point mutations that occur in critical positions in genes can significantly alter the functioning of a protein.

Polar body. A polar body is one of the products of female meiosis. During meiosis, male germ cells produce four sperm through two cell divisions of a single precursor cell. Female germ cells however, produce only one egg. In the first cell division of female meiosis the precursor cell, called the primary oocyte, divides to produce a secondary oocyte and a polar body. Female meiosis is paused at this time and does not resume until fertilization. At fertilization, the secondary oocyte divides to produce the egg and a second polar body. The polar bodies contain little besides the genetic material separated out during the cell division. Most of the contents of the cytoplasm of the primary oocyte are separated into the secondary oocyte and subsequently into the egg. The polar bodies are eventually lost while the egg provides the cytoplasm and combines its genetic material with that from the sperm.

Polymorphism. *See "mutation."*

Promoter. The promoter is the portion of a gene that guides the process and rate of synthesis of RNA. Mutations in the promoter region can affect the amount of RNA made from a gene. Such mutations can result in variations in the amount of a protein that gets made from a particular gene.

Protein. A protein is a molecule that performs specific functions within cells. Proteins can perform structural, regulatory, or enzymatic functions. Proteins are made up of amino acids and the amino acid sequence of a protein is specified by the DNA sequence of the gene for that protein. Defects in proteins due to mutations in DNA can alter the structure or function of cells, and such defects can result in genetic disease.

Rearrangement mutation. A rearrangement mutation is a mutation in which the DNA sequence of a gene is shuffled in some way. Rearrangements can flip segments of genes or chromosomes end for end or mix them in some other way. The consequences of the mutation depend upon the size, location, and nature of the rearrangement.

Recessive. Recessive is a term most often used when describing the physical effect of gene mutations or patterns of inheritance. Recessive gene mutations generally only exert a physical effect on the carrier in the absence of a normal gene.

Recombination. Recombination is a process that occurs during meiosis wherein segments are exchanged between the different chromosomes of a given pair. Recombination allows greater diversity among individuals by shuffling the combinations of gene sequences and changing the groups of genetic characteristics inherited by individuals in the next generation. Errors in recombination can result in mutations due to deletion, duplication, or rearrangement of genetic sequences.

Ribosome. Ribosomes are cellular structures that guide the manufacture of proteins. Ribosomes coordinate the conversion of RNA information into amino acids with the result of joining the individual amino acids together to create a protein. The amino acids incorporated into the new protein are specified by the sequence of the RNA through codons. *See "codon."*

RNA. RNA stands for ribonucleic acid. RNA is the molecule that serves as an intermediary between DNA and protein. This biochemical messenger is called messenger RNA (mRNA). mRNA is a copy of one strand of the DNA in a gene. mRNA carries the information from DNA in the nucleus to ribosomes in the cytoplasm for the manufacture of proteins. RNA is a less stable form of the genetic information than DNA, and there are slight chemical differences between the two molecules. RNA is single stranded. The four nucleotides used in RNA are adenine, cytosine, guanine, and uridine, or A, C, G, and U, respectively. *See "adenine," "cytosine," "guanine," "thymine," and "uridine."*

Somatic cell. Somatic cells are the cells of the body not destined to become germ cells.

Somatic cell nuclear transfer. Somatic cell nuclear transfer is the term used to describe one process by which an adult animal can be cloned. In somatic cell nuclear transfer, the nucleus of one somatic cell is transferred from the donor cell to another cell. For the purposes of cloning an entire animal, the donor nucleus is transferred to an egg cell from which the nucleus has been removed.

Somatic cell nuclear transfer is the method that was used to clone Dolly the sheep, the first cloned mammal, in Scotland in 1996. To create Dolly, the nucleus was removed from a sheep's egg cell. This enucleated egg was then fused with a somatic cell from another adult sheep. After fusion, the resulting embryo was implanted into a surrogate mother for gestation. Gestation resulted in the birth of Dolly. Somatic cell nuclear transfer has many applications for research beyond whole animal cloning.

Somatic mosaicism. Somatic mosaicism is the term used to describe the situation when a mutation is present in some but not in all of the somatic cells of an individual. Somatic mutations can occur when errors are made during duplication of the genome in mitosis or as a result of DNA damage. Many somatic mutations are probably clinically insignificant, but some mutations can result in disease if they are present in a large number of cells or if they disrupt a critical protein. Cancer is an example of a genetic disease caused by somatic mutations.

Sperm. The sperm is the germ cell produced by the male reproductive system for the formation of an embryo. The sperm contains little else besides one of each of the twenty-three chromosomes. At conception, the sperm fertilizes the egg and reconstitutes the total chromosome number of the egg cell to forty-six.

Teratogens. Teratogens are substances such as chemicals, drugs, viruses, bacteria, or medications that are capable of inducing birth defects. The effect of a teratogen on a fetus depends on several factors, including the time of exposure, the duration of the exposure, and the dosage of the exposure. Expectant mothers or women planning pregnancies should always ask about the teratogenic effects of parasites, bacteria, or viruses and any substances, drugs, or medications to which the fetus might be exposed. In addition, women should make sure their doctors are aware of the medications they take and ask about the teratogenic potential and appropriate doses of such medications during pregnancy.

Thymine. Thymine is one of the four nucleotides found in DNA. Thymine base pairs across the rungs of the DNA ladder with the nucleotide adenine. The nucleotide thymine is not found in RNA. In RNA, thymine is replaced by uridine. In the synthesis of RNA, adenine guides the addition of uridine to the growing nucleotide string. *See "adenine" and "uridine."*

Transcription. Transcription is the process by which DNA is copied into RNA. DNA is the permanent form of the genetic information and RNA is the temporary form of the genetic information used by ribosomes to construct proteins. RNA is chemically a little different from DNA and is a copy of one strand of the DNA molecule. RNA is single stranded. *See "DNA" and "RNA."*

Translation. Translation is the process by which the information contained in RNA is converted into protein. The information contained in the RNA molecule exists in three-nucleotide codons that are used to specify the order of amino acids incorporated into proteins. Translation occurs on ribosomes in the cytoplasm of the cell. *See "genetic code" and "ribosome."*

Translocation. A translocation occurs when an entire chromosome or part of a chromosome is moved from its normal position and attached onto another chromosome. When segments of two chromosomes are swapped for each other, the translocation is said to be a reciprocal translocation. Translocations that occur with no net loss of genetic material are said to be balanced. Translocation is different from recombination because recombination involves different chromosomes of a pair, such as an exchange between the two copies of chromosome 1. Translocation involves different chromosomes such as an exchange between chromosome 1 and chromosome 4.

Ultrasound. Ultrasound is a noninvasive diagnostic method that uses sound waves emitted from a transducer held against the body. The sound waves are reflected by internal organs and displayed on a video screen. Ultrasound can be used to examine the structure, size, and location of internal organs. Ultrasound can be used prenatally to examine a fetus or postnatally to study the organs inside the body. Prenatal use of ultrasound can detect heart defects or other structural or growth abnormalities. Postnatally, ultrasound can be used to image internal organs for detection of anomalies. Many such anomalies can be suggestive or diagnostic of genetic disease.

Uridine. Uridine is one of the four nucleotides found in RNA. The nucleotide uridine is not found in DNA. In DNA, uridine is replaced by thymine. In the synthesis of RNA, adenine guides the addition of uridine to the growing nucleotide string. *See "thymine."*

X inactivation. X inactivation is the process by which transcription from one of the X chromosomes in female cells is randomly switched off during development. There are some genes on the X chromosome that escape inactivation and are expressed from both copies of the X chromosome, but most genes are not expressed from the inactive X. The determination of which X is inactivated in a particular cell is usually random. Once inactivated, that X chromosome remains inactive in all the future mitotic products or daughter cells of that cell. Nonrandom X inactivation, where one X is active in a large proportion of cells, is thought to be one cause of X-linked recessive diseases in females. In these cases, if the predominantly active X carries a mutation, females can show symptoms of X-linked recessive disease. In individuals with additional X chromosomes, that is more than the usual number of two for females or one for males, each of the additional X chromosomes is generally inactivated.

Bibliography

Books

Biochemistry, 3rd ed., 1988. Lubert Stryer. W. H. Freeman and Co. New York

Clinical Genetics Handbook, 2nd ed., 1993. Arthur Robinson, and Mary G. Linden. Blackwell Scientific Publications, Inc. Cambridge, Mass.

DNA in Forensic Science: Theory, Techniques and Applications. 1990. J. Robertson, A. M. Ross, and L. A. Burgoyne, editors. Ellis Horwood, Ltd. New York

Essential Medical Genetics. 1991. J.M. Connor, and M.A. Ferguson-Smith. Blackwell Scientific Publications. Oxford

Genetics, 3rd ed., 1994. David L. Hartl. Jones and Bartlett Publishers. Boston

Hepatitis B Vaccines in Clinical Practice. 1993. Ronald W. Ellis, editor. Marcel Dekker, Inc. New York

Human Genetics, 1990. Gordon Edlin. Jones and Bartlett Publishers. Boston

Human Genetics: Problems and Approaches, 2nd ed., 1979. F. Vogel, and A. G. Motulsky. Springer-Verlag. Berlin

The Kings and Queens of England and Scotland, 1990. Plantagenet Somerset Fry. Grove Press. New York

Mendelian Inheritance in Man, 10th ed., 1992. Victor A. McKusick. The Johns Hopkins University Press. Baltimore

The Metabolic and Molecular Bases of Inherited Disease, 7th ed., 1995. Charles R. Scriver, Arthur L. Beaudet, William S. Sly, and David Valle, editors. McGraw-Hill, Inc. New York

Principles of Medical Genetics, 1990. Thomas D. Gelehrter, and Francis S. Collins. Williams and Wilkins. Baltimore

Smith's Recognizable Patterns of Human Malformation, 4th ed. 1988. K.L. Jones. W.B. Saunders Co. Philadelphia

Thompson and Thompson: Genetics in Medicine, 5th ed., 1991. Margaret W. Thompson, Roderick R. McInnes, and Huntington F. Willard. W.B. Saunders and Co., Harcourt Brace Jovanovich, Inc. Philadelphia

Articles, Conventional Media, and Internet

"Application of DNA Fingerprinting to Enforcement of Hunting Regulations in Ontario." E. Guglich, P. Wilson, and B. White. Journal of Forensic Sciences. Vol. 38, 1993, pp. 48–59

"ASHG Report: Statement on Informed Consent for Genetic Research." American Journal of Human Genetics. Vol. 59, 1996, pp. 471–474. http://www.faseb.org/genetics/ashg/policy/pol-25.htm

"Calls for cloning ban sell science short." Declan Butler, and Meredith Wadman. Nature. Vol. 386, March 6, 1997, pp. 8–9

"Cohen expected to identify Unknown Soldier from Vietnam War." CNN, June 30,1998.
http://cnn.com/US/9806/30/unknowns.01/index.html

"Development and production aspects of a recombinant yeast-derived hepatitis B vaccine." J. Stephenne. Vaccine. Vol. 8, supplement, 1990, pp. S69–S73

"DNA Fingerprinting." A. H. Carwood. Clinical Chemistry. Vol. 35, No. 9, 1989, pp. 1832–1837

"Ethical and Policy Issues of Human Cloning." Harold T. Shapiro. Science. Vol. 277, July 11, 1997, pp. 195–197

"Folic Acid and Pregnancy." Policy Statement from the American College of Medical Genetics.
http://www.faseb.org/genetics/acmg/pol-23.htm

"Forensic DNA Data Banking by State Crime Laboratories." Jean McEwen. American Journal of Human Genetics. Vol. 56, No. 6, 1995, pp. 1487–1492

"Gene discovery for crop improvement." G.B. Martin. Current Opinions in Biotechnology. Vol. 9, No. 2, April 1, 1998, pp. 220–226

"Gene therapy: Promises, problems and prospects." I.M. Verma and N. Somia. William A. Horton, editor. Growth, Genetics and Hormones. Vol. 14, No. 1, April 1998, pp. 12–13

"Gene therapy: Promises, problems and prospects." I.M. Verma and N. Somia. Nature. Vol. 389, No. 6648, September 18, 1997, pp. 239–242

"Genetic restriction of HIV-1 infection and progression to AIDS by a deletion allele of the CKR5 Structural Gene …" M. Dean, et al. *Science.* Vol. 273, No. 5283, September 27, 1996, pp. 1856–1862

"Homozygous defect in HIV-1 coreceptor accounts for resistance of some multiply-exposed individuals to HIV-1 infection." R. Liu, et al. *Cell.* Vol. 86, No. 3, August 9, 1996, pp. 367–377

"Human Factor IX Transgenic Sheep Produced by Transfer of Nuclei from Transfected Fetal Fibroblasts." A.E. Schnieke, et al. *Science.* Vol. 278, No. 5346, December 19, 1997, pp. 2130–2133

"Little Lamb, Who Made Thee." Sharon Begley. *Newsweek.* March 10, 1997. pp. 52–57

"Multiple chemical forms of hepatitis B surface antigen produced in yeast." D.E. Wampler, et al. *Proceedings of the National Academy of Sciences, USA.* Vol. 82, October 1985, pp. 6830–6834

"New Goals for the U.S. Human Genome Project: 1998-2003." F.S. Collins, et al., *Science.* Vol. 282, No. 5389, October 23, 1998, pp. 682–689

"Resistance to HIV-1 infection in caucasian individuals bearing mutant alleles of the CCR-5 chemokine receptor gene." M. Samson, et al. *Nature.* Vol. 382, No. 6593, August 22, 1996, pp. 722–725

"A Review of State Legislation on DNA Forensic Data Banking." Jean McEwen, and Philip Reilly. *American Journal of Human Genetics.* Vol. 54, No. 6, 1994, pp. 941–958

"Russia Delays Decision on Last Czar's Bones." Reuters, November 4, 1997. http://www.alexanderpalace.org/palace/newburial3.html

"Statement of the American Society of Human Genetics on Cystic Fibrosis Carrier Screening." American Journal of Human Genetics. Vol. 51, No. 6, 1992, pp. 1443–1444. http://www.faseb.org/genetics/ashg/policy/pol-10.htm

"Statement on Genetic Testing for Cystic Fibrosis." Policy Statement from the American College of Medical Genetics. http://www.faseb.org/genetics/acmg/pol-32.htm

"Tests Confirm Skeletons are Czar and his Family." Associated Press, January 26, 1998. http://www.alexanderpalace.org/palace/012698A.html

"Threatened Bans on Human Cloning Research Could Hamper Advances."
J. Stephenson. *Journal of the American Medical Association*. Vol.
277, No. 13, April 2, 1997, pp. 1023–1026

"The utility of DNA typing in forensic work." R. Chakraborty, and K. Kidd.
Science. Vol. 254, 1991, pp. 1735–1739

"Viable offspring derived from fetal and adult mammalian cells." I. Wilmut,
et al. *Nature*. Vol. 385, No. 6619, February 27, 1997, pp. 810–813

Internet Web Sites

The American Cancer Society.
http://cancer.org

The National Human Genome Research Institute.
http://www.nhgri.nih.gov

The Human Genome Organization.
http://hugo.gdb.org

The Human Genome Project.
http://www.ornl.gov/TechResources/Human_
Genome/tko/index.htm

Online Mendelian Inheritance in Man (OMIM™). Center for Medical
Genetics. Johns Hopkins University (Baltimore) and National
Center for Biotechnology Information. National Library of
Medicine (Bethesda, MD). 1997
http://www.ncbi.nlm.nih.gov/Omim

Index

Note: Page numbers in italics refer to tables or figures.

About the Author

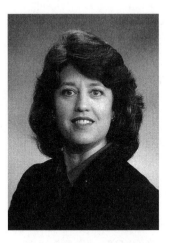

Raye Lynn Alford, Ph.D., is a graduate of Davidson College and Baylor College of Medicine. She is board certified in Clinical Molecular Genetics by the American Board of Medical Genetics and is a Fellow of the American College of Medical Genetics. She is a member of the American Society of Human Genetics and the Texas Genetics Society.

Dr. Alford has served on the faculty of Baylor College of Medicine as a laboratory scientist conducting genetic research and testing, and has coauthored numerous scientific articles reporting research results and reviewing topics in genetics. She has trained students and technicians in the laboratory, visited schools and medical conferences as a guest lecturer, and consulted with the Museum of Health and Medical Science in Houston, Texas, on the development of a genetics educational exhibit. Dr. Alford is Coordinator for Academic and Scientific Program Development in the Bobby R. Alford Department of Otorhinolaryngology and Communicative Sciences at Baylor College of Medicine.

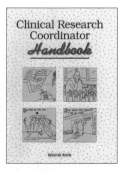
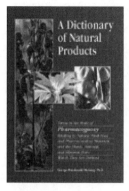
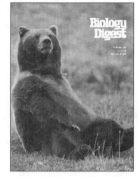